RESEARCH AND PERSPECTIVES IN ALZHEIMER'S DISEASE

Fondation Ipsen

Springer

Berlin
Heidelberg
New York
Barcelona
Hong Kong
London
Milan
Paris
Singapore
Tokyo

R. Mayeux Y. Christen (Eds.)

Epidemiology of Alzheimer's Disease: From Gene to Prevention

With 8 Figures and 21 Tables

Springer

Mayeux, Richard, MD
The Gertrude H. Sergievsky Center
630 West 168th Street
Columbia University
New York, NY 10032
USA

Christen, Y., Ph.D.
Fondation IPSEN
Pour la Recherche Thérapeutique
24, rue Erlanger
75781 Paris Cedex 16
France

ISSN 0945-6082
ISBN 3-540-65413-5 Springer-Verlag Berlin Heidelberg New York

Library of Congress Cataloging-in-Publication Data

Epidemiology of Alzheimer's : from gene to prevention / R. Mayeux, Y. Christen, eds. p. cm. – (Research and perspectives in Alzheimer's disease, ISSN 0945-6082) Includes bibliographical references and index. ISBN 3-540-65413-5 (alk. paper) 1. Alzheimer's disease – Epidemiology. I. Mayeux, Richard. II. Christen, Yves. III. Series. [DNLM: 1. Alzheimer Disease – epidemiology. 2. Alzheimer Disease – genetics. 3. Alzheimer Disease – prevention & control. WT 155 E64 1999] RA645.A49E65 1999 614.5'9831 – dc21 DNLM/DLC for Library of Congress

Production: PRO EDIT GmbH, D-69126 Heidelberg

Cover design: Design & Production, D-69121 Heidelberg

Typesetting: Mitterweger Werksatz GmbH, Plankstadt

SPIN: 10698813 27/3136 – 5 4 3 2 1 0 – Printed on acid-free paper

Preface

This volume contains the proceedings of the 14th Colloque Médecine et Recherche of the Fondation Ipsen pour la Recherche Thérapeutique devoted to Alzheimer's disease. It was held in Paris on May 25, 1998 and dedicated to the epidemiological study of this dementia, a very important issue because the incidence and prevalence of Alzheimer's disease rise exponentially with age.

Epidemiological findings not only confirm dementia as a major challenge for the coming years but also contribute defining risk factors, predicting and may be preventing this disease. All these issues have been tackled at the meeting in Paris and in the present book.

Y. C.

Contents

List of Contributors

Bots, M.L.
Department of Epidemiology & and Biostatistics, Erasmus University Medical School, PO Box 1738, 3000 DR Rotterdam, The Netherlands
and
Julius Center for Patient Oriented Research, University Medical Center, Heidelberglaan 100, 3584 CX Utrecht, The Netherlands

Brayne, C.
Department of Community Medicine-Institute of Public Health, Forvie Site-Robinson Way, Cambridge CB2 2SR, United Kingdom

Breteler, M. M. B.
Department of Epidemiology & and Biostatistics, Erasmus University Medical School, PO Box 1738, 3000 DR Rotterdam, The Netherlands

Dartigues, J.F.
INSERM U 330, Université de Bordeaux II, 146 rue Léo Saignat, 33076 Bordeaux Cedex, France

Dufouil, C.
INSERM Unit 360, Hôpital La Salpétrière, 75651 Paris Cédex 13, France

Evans, D.A.
Rush University and Rush Institute for Healthy Aging, 1645 W. Jackson Blvd., Chicago, IL 6061, USA

Fox, P.J.
Institute for Health and Aging, University of California, San Francisco, San Francisco, CA 94143–0612, USA

Ganguli, M.
University of Pittsburgh, Pittsburgh, PA 15213–3593, USA

Helmer, C.
INSERM U 330, Université de Bordeaux II, 146 rue Léo Saignat, 33076 Bordeaux Cedex, France

Henderson, V.W.
Department of Neurology, University of Southern California School of Medicine, 1420 San Pablo Street, Suite PMB-B105, Los Angeles, CA 90033, USA

Hendrie, H.C.
Department of Psychiatriy, Indiana University School of Medicine, 541 Clinical Drive, Room 298, Indianapolis, IN 46202–5111, USA

Hofman, A.
Department of Epidemiology & and Biostatistics, Erasmus University Medical School, PO Box 1738, 3000 DR Rotterdam, The Netherlands

Katzman, R.
Alzheimer's Disease Research Center, Department of Neurosciences, University of California, San Diego, La Jolla, CA 92093–0949, USA

Kawas, C.H.
Johns Hopkins University School of Medicine, 5501 Hopkins Bayview Circle, Room 1B.82, Baltimore, MD, 21224, USA

Khachaturian, Z.S.
Alzheimer's Association, Ronald & Nancy Reagan Research Institute, Chicago, IL 60611, USA

Letenneur, L.
INSERM U 330, Université de Bordeaux II, 146 rue Léo Saignat, 33076 Bordeaux Cedex, France

Mayeux, R.
The Gertrude H. Sergievsky Center, 630 West 168th Street, Columbia University, New York, NY 10032, USA

McGee, M.
MRC Biostatistics Unit-Institute of Public Health,
Forvie Site-Robinson Way, Cambridge CB2 2SR, United Kingdom

Ott, A.
Department of Epidemiology & and Biostatistics, Erasmus University Medical School, PO Box 1738, 3000 DR Rotterdam, The Netherlands
and
Department of Medical Microbiology, University Hospital Rotterdam, Dr. Molewaterplein 40, 3015 GD Rotterdam, The Netherlands

Radebaugh, T.S.
Alzheimer's Association, Ronald & Nancy Reagan Research Institute, Chicago, IL 60611, USA

Skoog, I.
Institute of Clinical Neuroscience, Department of Psychiatry, Sahlgrenska University Hospital, 413 45 Göteborg, Sweden

Slooter, A.J.C.
Department of Epidemiology & Biostatistics, Erasmus University Medical School, P.O. Box 1738, 3000 DR Rotterdam, The Netherlands

Tol, J.
Department of Epidemiology & Biostatistics, Erasmus University Medical School, P.O. Box 1738, 3000 DR Rotterdam, The Netherlands

van Duijn, C.M.
Department of Epidemiology & Biostatistics, Erasmus University Medical School, P.O. Box 1738, 3000 DR Rotterdam, The Netherlands

The World-Wide Impact of Dementia. Projections of Prevalance and Costs

R. Katzman[1] and P. J. Fox[2]

Summary

The prevalence of dementia and Alzheimer's disease (AD) is age-dependent, rising exponentially with increasing age. As a result the number of cases of dementia and Alzheimer's disease have risen this century, as the number of persons over age 65 has dramatically increased. During the next 50 years, the aging of the population will continue worldwide. According to 1996 United Nations projections, the population in the more developed countries will decline slightly from 1.19 to 1.16 billion between the years 2000 and 2050 but the number of individuals age 65 and over will increase from 169 million (14.2 % of the population) to 287 million (24.7 % of the population). Utilizing conservative prevalence estimates the number of individuals with dementia in developed countries will increase from 13.5 million in the year 2000 to 36.7 million in the year 2050, as an increasing number of very elderly survive. By 2050, incident cases of dementia in the United States will approach the number of incident cases of cancer. Formal and informal costs to care for patients with dementia will increase at least two-and-a-half-fold in constant dollars during this 50-year period.

During the same 50 years, increases in life expectancy in the less developed countries should mirror the increases that occurred in developed countries during the twentieth century. The percentage of the population age 65 and over will increase from 5 % to 13 % during this time period, exceeding 1.1 billion by the year 2050. There is less certainty as to the prevalence of dementia in less developed countries, but a reasonable estimate is that there will be over 65 million cases of dementia in 2050 and societal costs will increase more than eight-fold over current levels. Discovering how to prevent or delay the onset of AD and related dementing illnesses in order to reduce the prevalence of these disorders must be a high priority for all of our governments.

[1] Alzheimer Disease Research Center, Department of Neurosciences, University of California, San Diego, La Jolla, CA 92093-0949, USA.

[2] Institute for Health and Aging, University of California, San Francisco, San Francisco, CA 94143-0646, USA.

R. Mayeux / Y. Christen (Eds.)
Epidemiology of Alzheimer's Disease:
From Gene to Prevention

Introduction

Our objective is to estimate the world-wide impact of AD and other late life dementing disorders today and during the first half of the twenty-first century. On the assumption that current age-specific prevalence and incidence rates will remain unchanged, we can project the number of demented in the first half of the next century with some confidence in the more developed countries, but with trepidation in regard to the less developed countries.

The rise in life expectancy in the twentieth century will be matched by a rise in the number of elderly and hence in the number of those with dementia in the first 50 years of the twenty-first century. In 1900, life expectancy at birth was just under 50 years in what are now called the "more developed" countries, the industrialized countries. There were so few elderly that, from a public health point of view, "senile dementia" was appropriately ignored. In the year 2000, life expectancy at birth will reach 75.3 years in the more developed countries – a gain of 25 years in one century, or three months every calendar year. The direct consequence of this remarkable increase in longevity and the increase in the number of very elderly during the twentieth century is that AD and other late life dementing disorders have become major causes of morbidity and mortality in the developed countries. By a very conservative United Nations (UN) estimate, life expectancy at birth will continue to increase but at a slower pace and will reach 80.9 years in the year 2050 in the more developed countries (Table 1). Yet during this period, the proportion of the population age 65 and over in the more developed countries will almost double (Table 2). The number of individuals with AD and other dementing illnesses will increase at a faster rate, since the proportion of those age 85 or over, who are at very high risk for developing dementia, will

Table 1. Life expectancy at birth. Median variant projections (UN 1996)

	1950–1955	1970–1975	2000–2005	2020–2025	2040–2050
World total	46.5	57.9	66.9	72.1	76.3
More developed[a]	66.5	71.2	75.3	78.3	80.8
Less developed[b]	40.1	54.7	65.1	70.8	75.5
Specific Countries:					
United States	69.0	71.3	77.4	79.7	81.5
Canada	69.1	73.1	79.4	81.2	82.9
France	66.5	72.4	79.4	81.1	83.0
Italy	66.0	72.1	79.2	81.4	83.3
Sweden	71.8	74.7	79.4	81.6	83.4
United Kingdom	69.2	72.0	77.9	79.9	81.8
China	40.8	63.2	71.0	74.6	77.9
Japan	63.9	73.3	80.3	81.8	83.6

a) More developed = North America, Japan, Europe and Australia/New Zealand.
b) Less developed = Asia (excluding Japan), Africa, Latin America and Caribbean, Melanesia, Micronesia, and Polynesia.

Table 2. United Nations population projections. Estimates of population 65 plus

	2000			2025			2050		
In millions:	Population	65+[c]	Population 65+	Population	65+[c]	Population 65+	Population	65+[c]	Population 65+
World total	6091	0.068	414	8039	0.10	804	9367	0.151	1414
More developed[a]	1187	0.142	169	1220	0.20	244	1162	0.247	287
Less developed[b]	4904	0.05	245	6819	0.081	552	8205	0.138	1132
In thousands:									
Canada	30679	0.126	3866	36385	0.205	7459	36352	0.245	8906
France	59061	0.162	9568	60393	0.225	13588	58370	0.264	15410
Italy	57194	0.177	10123	51744	0.256	13246	42092	0.357	15027
Sweden	8898	0.167	1486	9511	0.216	2054	9574	0.232	2221
United Kingdom	58336	0.158	9217	59535	0.203	12086	58733	0.232	13626
United States	277825	0.124	34450	332481	0.183	60844	347543	0.212	73679
China	1276301	0.067	85512	1480430	0.122	180612	1516664	0.192	291199
Japan	126428	0.165	20861	121348	0.259	31429	109546	0.304	33302

a) More developed = North America, Japan, Europe and Australia/New Zealand.
b) Less developed = Asia (excluding Japan), Africa, Latin America and Caribbean, Melanesia, Micronesia, and Polynesia.
c) Proportion of population over 65.

increase almost four-fold during this period. Evans (1990) has shown that if the age-specific prevalence figures obtained in the survey of Alzheimer's disease carried out in the 1980s in East Boston, Massachusetts, are projected to the United States population distribution in 2050 (middle series, US Census Bureau), the number of individuals with AD will reach 14.5 million in 2050, which is triple the current number.

Demography of Aging

Projections of total population and number of those age 65 and older in the years 2000, 2025 and 2050 are shown in Table 2. This table is based upon the middle series of the 1996 Revision of the United Nations "World Population Prospects," which takes into account the falling fertility and mortality rates as well as the impact of AIDS. In our table we have included the data for the entire world, for the "more developed countries," which are defined by the United Nations as the countries in North America and Europe, Japan and Australia/New Zealand, for the remaining "less developed countries," and for eight specific countries.

Fertility in more developed countries has now fallen below the replacement rate so that the total population of the more developed countries will actually decrease from 1.19 billion in the year 2000 to 1.16 billion in 2050, yet the population age 65 and older will increase from 14.2 % of the total population in 2000 to 24.7 % of the total population in 2050. During the same period, the proportion of those age 85 or over will increase almost four-fold to reach 6 % of the total population. If one assumes that there will be no change in the age-specific prevalence rates between the years 2000 and 2050, the number of persons with dementia in the more developed countries will increase two-and-a-half-fold due to the aging of their populations over this interval.

Among the less developed countries, a rapid growth in life expectancy is well underway in Asia and Latin America but is only now beginning to catch up with the gains experienced in developed countries. In the less developed countries, the total population will increase from 4.9 billion in the year 2000 to 8.2 billion in 2050; the percentage of those age 65 and over will increase from 5 % to 13 % during the next 50 years, exceeding 1.1 billion by the year 2050.

Prevalence and Incidence of Dementia and Alzheimer's Disease Rise Exponentially with Age

Alzheimer's disease – which accounts for three-fifths to three-quarters of those with dementia – and other dementing disorders are prototypic age-dependent disorders whose prevalence and incidence rise exponentially with increasing age. Analyzing data from 22 pre-1986 studies of dementia, Jorm et al. (1987) found that despite marked differences in prevalence rates between the studies, there was a consistent exponential relationship between prevalence rates and age across these studies, such that the rates doubled with every 5.1 years of age.

Almost identical results were obtained in 10 additional prevalence studies published after 1985 (summarized by Katzman and Kawas 1994).

A major problem in projecting the number of demented individuals is the wide discrepancy in age-specific prevalence reported between studies. Yet the exponential rise in the prevalence with age within each study remains consistent. Jorm et al. (1988) proposed that projections of future numbers of persons with dementia or AD be expressed as a percentage rise, which can be easily obtained by applying the exponential equation relating age-specific prevalence and age to the changes in the age composition of the population during the period to be studied. At one extreme, they projected a rise in the prevalence of dementia of 100 % in the United States between 1980 and 2025, and of 215 % in Japan, whose population is aging most rapidly.

Recently, data on follow-up surveys of the incidence of new cases of dementia and AD in several of these populations have been reported. Incidence also increases exponentially with age, doubling with every five years of increase in age after age 65 (Hebert et al. 1995; Brookmeyer et al. 1998).

Variations in Prevalence Rates between Studies

Epidemiological studies of the prevalence of dementia and AD in persons age 65 and older have shown wide variation, from 4 % to 12 %. In part this variation can be attributed to variations in population age structure between communities, but there are also marked differences in age-specific prevalence rates between studies. While about three-fourths of this variation can be attributed to differences in criteria and methodology (Corrada et al. 1995), other factors such as educational level, ethnicity and differential mortaliy in diverse populations may play a role. The contrast in methodologies used is best illustrated by comparison of the age-specific prevalence estimates made in the East Boston and Framingham surveys.

Age-specific prevalence rates for AD estimated in the Framingham study (Bachmann et al. 1992; 1993) were about one-sixth that observed in East Boston (Evans et al. 1989). The two communities are located within 30 miles of each other in eastern Massachusetts; both are almost entirely white communities with a significant portion of their populations of Italian-American derivation, although the educational and economic level of the population is lower in East Boston. However, the two studies were carried out very differently. East Boston was a total community study in which the investigators clinically investigated a stratified subset of subjects, sampled upon the basis of their scores on a sensitive test for a specific cognitive decline seen early in AD, a test for delayed recall (the "East Boston" story). These investigators based their diagnoses on clinical evidence of cognitive decline. The Framingham study was carried out in the context of a longitudinal study of risk factors for cardiovascular and cerebrovascular diseases that had been ongoing for several decades. These investigators were interested in identifying risk factors for AD and sought unequivocal cases. Hence they used the 23/24 cut-off score on the Mini Mental State Examination (MMSE; Folstein) as their screening tool and required demonstration of a moderately severe degree of cognitive and functional loss for diagnosis of AD and dementia.

Corrada et al.'s (1995) analysis of the discrepancies of age-specific rates of dementia and AD reported in different studies indicated that some of the methodological sources of variation between studies are epidemiological:ascertainment of a sample rather than the total population, inclusion of both urban and rural populations, and failure to adjust for false negatives. Another set of factors was related to the criteria required for the diagnosis of dementia, i.e. how mild were the cases to be included. The remaining factors were related to the differential diagnosis of dementing illnesses, particularly AD, vascular dementia, and dementia due to other illnesses, and whether the investigators used or did not use laboratory tests, CT scans and the Hachinski score.

These latter sources of variation point to the difficulties inherent in epidemiological studies in accurately differentiating AD and vascular dementia. There is now evidence from clinical-pathological evaluation of diagnoses in patients who have been intensively evaluated in specialized dementia centers that while the positive diagnosis of AD based on the DSMIII or DSMIII-R and the NINDCS/ADRDA criteria (McKhann et al. 1984) achieves an accuracy of 85–90 %, the accuracy of diagnosis of the second most common form of dementia, vascular dementia, is sometimes as low as 50 % (Galasko et al. 1994). This is in part due to the lack of specificity of the Hachinski scale (Rosen et al. 1980) and in part due to our current clinical inability to differentiate between AD with stroke associated with amyloid angiopathy, a manifestation of AD, in hypertensive individuals (Olichney et al. 1995) and primary atherosclerotic multi-infarct dementia. Moreover, the prevalence studies carried out in the 1980s and 1990s did not take into account recently described criteria for vascular dementia (Chui et al. 1992; Roman et al. 1993) or recognition of and development of diagnostic criteria for non-AD degenerative dementias, including the fronto-temporal dementias and dementia with Lewy bodies. Because of these diagnostic confounds that are inherent in the existing epidemiological prevalence studies, we have chosen to utilize data on the age-specific prevalence rates of dementia rather than of AD in our projections.

Furthermore, if we are to project costs attributable to dementing disorders, we need to select age-specific prevalence rates for dementia based upon studies that have surveyed both community-residing and institutionalized residents of a community. This criterion eliminates longitudinal studies such as the Framingham survey and practice-based studies such as those from the Mayo Clinic in Rochester, Minnesota (Kokmen et al. 1996), which was based on clinic and physician practices. Among the community studies carried out since 1980 that include both community and institutionalized residents, the East Boston survey utilized a delayed recall test, a sensitive measure of early cognitive change in AD and dementia.

Most of the other epidemiological studies that included both community-residing and institutionalized persons utilized criteria for the diagnosis of dementia based upon DSMIII (American Psychiatric Association 1980) or the

1987 version, DSMIII-R, requiring unequivocal evidence of functional decline. Among these studies the most common screening test used was the Mini-Mental Status Examination (Folstein et al. 1975) with a cut-off score of 23/24 (30 is the best possible score) or its equivalent [such as a score of 77/78 (out of 100) on the 3MS].

The cut-off score of 23/24 on the Mini Mental State Examination (MMSE) had been shown by Folstein et al. (1975) and confirmed by Anthony et al. (1982) to differentiate patients with dementia from normals and from those with depression or other psychiatric conditions. This cut-off value has served to insure that patients who are selected for drug trials or case-control studies are truly demented. This approach has increased the accuracy of diagnoses (Galasko et al. 1994) and reduced the number of false positive subjects in epidemiological surveys, significantly reducing the number of clinical evaluations and hence the cost. However, it results in false negatives.

Our understanding of the clinical aspects of AD and other dementing illnesses has improved with the recognition that impairment of delayed recall and reduction in verbal fluency are accurate markers of very mildly impaired patients despite scores on the MMSE well above 23. The diagnosis of dementia in very mildly impaired subjects with MMSE scores of 24 or more at first examination has now become routine in many specialized centers. For example, at the Alzheimer Disease Research Center at the University of California, San Diego, the percentage of patients diagnosed as demented on initial examination who had an MMSE score ≥ 24 increased from 14 % in 1985 to 55 % in 1995. The accuracy of the diagnosis of dementia in a series of 110 of these research subjects was 94 %, based upon subsequent follow-up examinations including autopsies in 38 patients. Since the East Boston prevalence and incidence surveys used a sensitive measure of delayed recall rather than the MMSE to identify patients with dementia, it is likely that their prevalence data differ from studies using the MMSE 23/24 as a screening tool, because of the East Boston survey's ability to identify the very mildly impaired. One could argue that the East Boston prevalence and incidence figures include very mildly demented individuals not identified by the usual epidemiological approach and more accurately identify the totality of demented subjects. But the societal and fiscal costs of these mildly impaired patients have not yet been studied. To determine costs we need to use available cost surveys and match them with suitable age-specific prevalence numbers. Therefore for our purposes, the age-specific prevalence data obtained by studies using this standard MMSE cut-off are appropriate.

Hofman et al. (1991) and Rocca et al. (1991) reported the results of the EURODEM collaborative reanalysis of the prevalence of AD and dementia. Out of 23 European data sets available, they identified six that met other criteria and included both community and institutional subjects, constituting a sample of 5671 persons over the age of 60, including 1640 age 80 and over. All but one of these six selected surveys used the MMSE 23/24 cut-off score for subject screening prior to being evaluated for dementia. A similar but larger, multi-site survey was carried out by the Canadian Study of Health and Aging in nine Canadian provinces in 1990 to 1992 using a score of 78 (out of 100) on the 3MS mental status test as their screening instrument, a score similar to the 23/24 on the MMSE. The Canadian study included 9008 subjects age 65 and older in the comunity and 1225 in institutions. Moreover, there were 1858 subjects 85 years and older. Their data on the very elderly are of particular importance since the EURODEM analysis included only 107 subjects age 90–94 and none age 95 or over, whereas the Canadian study included 371 age 90–94 and 104 in the 95 years and older sample (Canadian Study of Health and Aging 1994; Ebly et al. 1994). It is striking that the prevalence of dementia in the Canadian sample of subjects age 95 and older was 58 %, the number to which the Jorm et al. (1987) semi-log plot of dementia prevalence vs age projects, although in the original Jorm data set there were no subjects in that advanced age group to include in their analysis. Since the most rapidly rising portion of the population in the next century is these very elderly, we will therefore use the age-specific prevalence figures from the Canadian Study of Health and Aging in our calculations.

Projections of the Prevalence of Dementia

Table 3 shows our projections of the number of demented subjects in the more developed countries in the years 2000, 2025 und 2050 and for six individual developed countries – Canada, France, Italy, Sweden, United Kingdom and the United States – for which there are data for the formal or informal costs of care, as well as for China and Japan. We also provide projections in regard to the number

Table 3. Projected numbers of cases of dementia (in thousands)

	2000	2025[a]	2050[a]
More developed[b]	13520	21228	36736
Less developed[c]	8575	25392	67920
World-wide	22095	46620	104656
Canada	309	649	1140
France	765	1182	1972
Italy	810	1152	1973
Sweden	119	179	284
United Kingdom	737	1051	1744
United States	2756	5293	9431
China[d]	3934	8308	23290
Japan	1669	2718	4263

a) Population projections are the 1998 Middle Series (United Nations).

b) Prevalence estimates in developed countries based upon Canadian Study of Health and Aging adjusted for changing population structure in years 2025 and 2050 (Canadian Study of Health and Aging Working Group 1994; Ebly et al. 1994).

c) Prevalence estimates for less developed countries on assumption that 2025 age distribution of the elderly will be equivalent to that of China in year 2000, based upon projected life expectancies.

d) Prevalence estimates for China based upon Shanghai data and then adjusted for projected changes in Chinese age structure (Zhang et al. 1990).

of cases of dementia in these years in China and Japan, countries for which detailed data on projected population structure are available. In the case of China, the age distribution of their elderly in 2050 will approach that of the United States today, whereas Japan will have the highest percentage worldwide of those over the age of 85.

The 1987 Shanghai survey of dementia (Zhang et al. 1990) meets the criteria we have used above; it was a community study using DSMIII criteria and the MMSE as a survey tool. Cut-off points in selecting subjects for a detailed clinical evaluation were 23/24 on the MMSE for those with six years or more of formal education, 21/22 for those with less than six years, and 19/20 for those who had received no education, based on a prior pilot study (Katzman et al. 1988), with additional evaluation of a 5 % sample of subjects who were above cut-off. We now use the Shanghai age-specific prevalence figure and data available to us on the projected age distribution of the over 65 Shanghai population in the next half century to project the number of demented persons in China in the years 2000 and 2025.

Estimates of the number of dementia patients in the less developed world today can only be an arbitrary guess since there is little or no information available outside of Southeast Asia. We have used the Shanghai over 65 age distribution, adjusting for life expectancy, to provide a basis for late-life age distribution in the less developed countries. However, applying the age-specific prevalence rates for dementia obtained in Southeast Asia to the remainder of the less developed world is fraught with uncertainty. Several studies have been conducted in Latin America but not yet published; initial indications are that these will have prevalence rates reasonably close to those of Shanghai. The one published survey from India (Shaji et al. 1996) reports an overall prevalence of dementia about 25 % lower than the Shanghai survey. The one published study from sub-Saharan Africa (Nigeria; Hendrie et al. 1994) reported prevalence rates very much lower than those in Shanghai. The length of survival of dementia patients in Nigeria is unknown but differences in survival may not explain the differences in prevalence (Hendrie, personal communication). It is interesting that the data in regard to the prevalence of dementia observed in Nigeria differ from the prevalence of dementia in Afro-Americans in Indianapolis, Indiana, although the two studies used similar methods (Hendrie et al. 1994). Hence the application of the Shanghai prevalence estimates to less developed countries such as India, Middle Eastern countries or African countries is arbitrary and may overstate the magnitude of the current problem.

Incidence of Dementia

Epidemiological studies of the prevalence of dementia and AD in those age 65 and older have shown wide variation, from 4 to 12 %, as discussed above. In contrast to the prevalence surveys, many of the reported incidence studies show a much narrower range of variation in age-specific incidence rates. Recent incidence data from Hisayama (Ueda et al. 1992; Yoshitake et al. 1995), North Man-

Table 4. Comparison of projected incident cases of AD and invasive cancer (in thousands)

	1996	2050
Cancer, invasive	1,272	2,763
AD[a]	750	2,476

[a)] Projection based upon East Boston age-specific incidence rates (Hebert et al. 1996).

hattan (Tang et al. 1998) and the Baltimore Longitudinal Survey of Dementia (Brookmeyer et al. 1998) are similar to those of East Boston (Hebert et al. 1995). Surprisingly, the incidence rates in the East Boston and Shanghai surveys (Yu et al., in preparation) are similar. If the adjusted age-specific incidence figures obtained in the Shanghai survey are applied to the 1996 US population distribution, the annual incidence rate would be 2.1 % per year in those age 65 and over, almost identical to the 2.2 % per year obtained if one utilizes the age-specific incidence rates reported in East Boston (Hebert et al. 1995). The differences in prevalence found between Shanghai and East Boston may be attributable in part to the shorter life expectancy of demented subjects in Shanghai.

If the age-specific incidence estimates of AD in East Boston are projected to the US population in 2050, the number of new or incident cases of AD will be 2.5 million per year. This number is close to the 2.7 million new cases of cancer projected in the United States in 2050 (Table 4). These projections assume that there will be no progress in preventing or delaying the onset of either disease. If current prospects of new therapeutic approaches to cancer achieve even modest success, the dementing illnesses may become the second most important set of diseases by the middle of the next century.

The Economic Burden of Dementia

When considering the estimation of the economic burden of AD cross-nationally, difficulties in comparisons arise due to substantial methodological variations that exist in published reports, as well as differences in the structure of health and long-term care systems that contribute to the overall costs of caring for people with AD and related dementias. Some studies estimate average per capita or national costs based on a set of assumptions applied to national data (Gray and Fenn 1993; Hay and Ernst 1987; Ernst and Hay 1994; Wimo et al. 1997; Huang et al. 1988), whereas others rely on the collection of primary data from samples of demented people which vary in size from tens to thousands of patients (Østbye and Crosse 1994; Hu et al. 1986; Souêtre et al. 1995; Stommel et al. 1994; Weinberger et al. 1993; Rice et al. 1993; Max et al. 1995; Cavallo and Fattore 1997; Welch et al. 1992).

To complicate matters further, studies consider different cost components. While almost all published studies available in English consider both direct (i.e., costs that result in actual monetary expenditures, such as paying for a home care worker) and indirect (i.e., costs that do not result in actual monetary expenditures such as the time a wife spends helping her demented spouse) costs, the components of each differ to varying degrees from study to study. While most studies include estimates of hospital care, physician visits, medications, and institutional care as part of direct cost calculations, a much smaller proportion include dementia-related research or diagnostic costs. Most studies also include indirect costs associated with valuing unpaid caregiver time assisting demented persons, but a much smaller proportion include costs associated with premature mortality and lost producitivity attributable to AD and related dementias. Matters are complicated even further in that some studies focus specifically on persons with AD whereas others include people with multiple types of dementing disorders. In spite of these analytical differences, these studies provide the only published data upon which to base national cost estimates for the care of people with AD in these countries.

To estimate the per capita costs in 1998 dollars, we identified the per capita average annual cost of care for people with AD or a related dementia. If the total was not reported in US dollars, we made the conversion based on 1996 foreign exchange rates. We then inflated the average to 1998 dollars using the particular nations's five-year (1992–96) average inflation rate. To estimate total costs per country, we then multiplied the per capita average by the estimated number of cases of AD for the years 2000, 2025, and 2050. Table 5 displays the annual per patient cost estimates for these six countries and projects total costs as well as percentage increases for the first half of the twenty-first century.

When projecting such costs into the future, we have made the following simplifying assumptions:

- Costs attributable to people with dementia are the same as those attributable specifically to people with AD.
- Calculated annual per person cost averages are constant across all segments of the population with AD in a particular country.
- The total social costs of caring for people with AD in institutions is the same as for people with AD who reside in their homes, although there is substantial variation as to the proportion of total costs accounted for by direct and indirect elements.
- The per capita costs will be the same in 2000, 2025, and 2050 as they are estimated to be in 1998.

Table 5. Cost of dementia care: estimates for selected countries in first half of the twenty-first century

Country	Annual per patient cost estimate (1998 US$)	US$ in billions[a]			Increase 2000–2025 (%)	Increase 2025–2050 (%)	50-year total increase (%)
		2000	2025	2050			
Canada	11,210	3.4	7.3	12.8	115	75	276
England	15,454	4.7	6.8	11.2	45	65	138
France	64,800	11.8	18.3	30.5	55	67	158
Italy	15,187	52.5	74.7	124.6	42	67	137
Sweden	6,452	1.8	2.7	4.3	50	59	139
United States	40,622	111.9	215.0	383.1	92	78	242

[a)] 1998 dollars.

Projected Estimates of the Cost of Caring for People with Alzheimer's Disease:

England

The only English study of the costs of caring for people with AD (Gray and Fenn 1993) estimated the annual cost in England at £ 1.039 billion. This study did not include an imputed value for unpaid informal caring services provided by family members. Other studies have shown that this accounts for the greatest portion of the costs of caring for people with AD, ranging from a high of 76 % (Huang et al. 1988) to a low of 36 % (Souêtre et al. 1995) of total care costs. As such, the cost calculations for the UK will be substantially lower than for other countries.

To estimate the cost of informal care for England, we took the midpoint of the published ranges as the estimated proportion of total costs accounted for by unpaid caregiving assistance. This yields a figure of 56 % of total costs attributable to informal care provision, which is very close to the 51 % estimated for the US by Ernst and Hay (1987). Applying this percentage to the Gray and Fenn (1993) 1990–91 cost estimate of £ 1.039 billion yields an estimated total cost of £ 2.36 billion pounds for England. Assuming a 2.7 % average annual inflation rate (18.9 % total inflation from 1992–98) yields a total cost estimate of £ 2.81 billion. Using an exchange rate of £ 0.641 per dollar ($ 1.56 per pound), the total 1998 cost of care estimate for England is $ 4.4 billion.

Given the estimated number of prevalent cases of AD in the 65 years and older population in England (8.7 % of those 65 years and older or 681,943 people with AD) and dividing that by the total estimated costs yields a per capita care annual cost estimate of approximately $ 6,452. Using this estimate and assuming that the per capita cost for England reflects the UK, we applied the figure to the projected prevalence of AD in the UK in the years 2000, 2025, and 2050 and we arrived at an annual AD burden of approximately $ 4.8 billion, $ 6.8 billion, and $ 11.2 billion, respectively.

France

The 1991 per capita annual costs of AD in France have been estimated to be approximately $ 13,556 (Souêtre et al. 1995). Applying a 2 % average annual inflation rate (14 % total from 1992–98) results in a 1998 estimate of $ 15,454. Applying this per person estimate to projected prevalence figures for 2000, 2025, and 2050 yields economic cost estimates for France of $ 11.8 billion, $ 18.3 billion, and $ 30.5 billion, respectively.

Canada

The 1991 per capita annual costs of AD in Canada have been estimated to be approximately $ 13,900 Canadian (Østbye and Crosse 1994). Using an exchange rate of $ 1.37 and applying a 1.5 % annual inflation rate (10.5 % total from

1992–98) results in a 1998 estimate of $ 11,210. Applying this per person estimate to projected prevalence figures for 2000, 2025, and 2050 yields economic cost estimates for Canada of $ 3.5 billion, $ 7.3 billion, and $ 12.8 billion, respectively.

Italy

The 1995 per capita annual costs of non-medical care for people with AD in the Lombardy region of Italy have been estimated to be approximately $ 52,954 (Cavallo and Fattore 1997). Applying a 4.6 % average annual inflation rate (13.8 % total for 1996–1998) results in a 1998 estimate of $ 60,261. Since this estimate does not include medical care associated with the care of people with AD, we estimated from other published studies what those costs may be based on the proportion of total costs accounted for by medical care. Medical care costs for this group have been reported to account for between a high of 11 % (Souêtre et al. 1995) and a low of 3.4 % (Østbye and Crosse 1994) based on studies of the costs of caring of people with AD in other countries. Using the midpoint of the range, we estimate medical care costs to constitute approximately 7 % of total costs. Applying this estimate to the present study yields a total annual per capita cost estimate of approximately $ 64,800. Applying this per person estimate to projected prevalence figures for 2000, 2025, and 2050 yields economic cost estimates for Italy of $ 52.5 billion, $ 74.7 billion, and $ 124.6 billion, respectively.

Sweden

The 1991 per capita annual costs of AD in Sweden have been estimated to be approximately $ 13,003 (Wimo et al. 1997). Applying a 2.4 % annual inflation rate (16.8 % total from 1992–98) results in a 1998 estimate of $ 15,187. Applying this per person estimate to projected prevalence figures for 2000, 2025, and 2050 yields economic cost estimates for Sweden of $ 1.8 billion, $ 2.7 billion, and $ 4.3 billion, respectively.

United States

Per capita annual costs of AD in the US have been estimated to range from a low of $ 11,261 (Huang et al. 1988) to a high of $ 52,600 (Weinberger et al. 1993). Converting these estimates into 1998 dollars assuming a 2.8 % average annual inflation rate yields an annual range of from $ 15,360 to $ 65,885. Using the midpoint of this range yields an annual estimated per person cost of $ 40,622. Applying this per person estimate to projected prevalence figures for 2000, 2025, and 2050 yields economic cost estimates for the US of $ 111.9 billion, $ 215.0, and $ 383.1 billion, respectively.

Discussion

Because of different cost estimation methodologies used, as well as the varying structure of the health and long-term care systems in the countries for which AD cost studies are available, substantial variations exist when examining per capital-annual costs associated with the care of people with AD. Where practical, we have attempted to estimate some costs that may have not been accounted for in the original research. For example, we estimated the cost of informal care in England and the cost of medical care services in Italy, both of which were excluded from consideration in the respective studies. The adjustments are relatively crude, but they help to improve comparability of the estimates across studies.

Because of the wide variation in per capita cost estimates, it is more instructive to compare the increase in total costs as the aging of the populations occur. As shown in Table 5, for all nations considered, the estimated increase in costs associated with the care of people with AD will rise dramatically in the next 50 years from a high 276 % increase in Canada to a low 137 % increase in Italy. The "true" costs of caring for people with AD in the countries is difficult to compare because of:

1) the inclusion of different cost elements;
2) the use of different values to impute an economic value to non-paid care provision;
3) consistent lack of data on costs associated with caring for demented people in institutional versus community-resident living arrangements;
4) cross-national differences in the structure and financing of health and long-term care; and
5) problems inherent in attempting to calculate the costs of a demented population's care based on studies consisting of nonrepresentative samples.

In spite of these difficulties, it is clear that the rough estimates we have derived from published studies of the cost of caring for people with AD, without exception, indicate a substantial increase in the costs of caring for increasingly large numbers of people with AD and related dementias.

Acknowledgments

Supported in part by the National Institute on Aging (AGO5131-15) and the State of California (97-10931). We thank Alicia Booth and Sue Johnson for their assistance.

References

American Psychiatric Association Task Force on Nomenclature and Statistics (ed) (1980) Diagnostic and statistical manual of mental disorders (DSM-III) 3rd Ed. American Psychiatric Association, Washington, DC

American Psychiatric Association Task Force on Nomenclature and Statistics (ed) (1987) Diagnostic and statistical manual of mental disorders, revised (DSM-III-R) 3rd Revised Ed. American Psychiatric Association, Washington, DC

Anthony JC, LeResche L, Unaiza N, Von Korff MR, Folstein MF (1982) Limits of the 'Mini-Mental State' as a screening test for dementia and delirium among hospital patients. Psychol Med 12:397–408

Bachman DL, Wolf PA, Linn R, Knoefel JE, Cobb J, Belanger A, D'Agostino RB, White LR (1992) Prevalence of dementia and probable senile dementia of the Alzheimer type in the Framingham Study. Neurology 42:115–119

Bachmann DL, Wolf PA, Linn RT, Knoefel JE, Cobb JL, Belanger AJ, White LR, D'Agostino RB (1993) Incidence of dementia and probable Alzheimer's disease in general population: the Framingham study. Neurology 43:515–519

Brookmeyer R, Gray S, Kawas C (1998) Projections of Alzheimer's disease in the United States and the public health impact of delaying disease onset. Am J Public Health 88:1337–1342

Canadian Study of Health and Aging Working Group (1994) Canadian Study of Health and Aging: study methods and prevalence of dementia. Can Med Assoc J 150:899–912

Cavallo MC, Fattore G (1997) The economic and social burden of Alzheimer disease on families in the Lombardy region of Italy. Alzheimer Dis Assoc Disorders 11:184–190

Chui HC, Victoroff JI, Margolin D, Jagust W, Shankle R, Katzmann R (1992) Criteria for the diagnosis of ischemic vascular dementia proposed by the State of California Alzheimer Disease Diagnostic and Treatment Centers. Views & Reviews. Neurology 42:473–480

Corrada M, Brookmeyer R, Kawas C (1995) Sources of variability in prevalence rates of Alzheimer's disease. Int J Epidemiol 24:1000–1005

Ebly EM, Parhad IM, Hogan DB, Fung TS (1994) Prevalence and types of dementia in the very old: results, from the Canadian Study of Health and Aging. Neurology 44:1593–1600

Ernst RL, Hay JW (1994) The US economic and social costs of Alzheimer's disease revisited. Am J Public Health 84:1261–1264

Evans DA (1990) Estimated prevalence of Alzheimer's disease in the United States. Milbank Quart 68:267–289

Evans DA, Funkenstein HH, Albert MS, Scherr PA, Cook NR, Chown MJ, Hebert LE, Hennekens CH, Taylor JO (1989) Prevalence of Alzheimer's disease in a community population of older persons – Higher than previously reported. JAMA 262:2551–2556

Folstein MF, Folstein SE, McHugh PR (1975) "Mini-mental state." A practical method for grading the cognitive state of patients for the clinician. J Psych Res 12:189–198

Galasko D, Hansen LA, Katzmann R, Wiederholt W, Masliah E, Terry R, Hill LR, Lessin P, Thal LJ (1994) Clinical-neuropathological correlations in Alzheimer's disease and related dementias. Arch Neurol 51(9):888–895

Gray A, Fenn P (1993) Alzheimer's disease: the burden of the illness in England. Health Trends 25: 31–37

Hay JW, Ernst RL (1987) The economic costs of Alzheimer's disease. Am J Public Health 77:1169–1175

Hebert LE, Scherr PA, Beckett LA, Alberts MS, Pilgrim DM, Chown MJ, Funkenstein HH, Evans DA (1995) Age-specific incidence of Alzheimer's disease in a community population. JAMA 273:1354–1359

Hendrie H, Osuntokun B, Hall K, Ogunniyi A, Farlow M, Gurege O, Unverzagt F, Baiyewu O, Hui S (1994) A comparison of the prevalence of dementia and Alzheimer's disease in community dwelling residents of Ibadan, Nigeria, and Indianapolis, USA Neurobiol Aging 15 (suppl 1):S42

Hofman A, Rocca WA, Amaducci L (1991) A collaborative study of the prevalence of dementia in Europe: The EURODEM findings. In: Gottfries CG, Levy SR, Clinche G, Trirsmans L (Eds) Diagnostic and therapeutic assessments in Alzheimer's disease. Wrightson Biomedical Publishing Ltd., pp 100–116

Hu T, Huang L, Cartwright W (1986) Evaluation of the costs of caring for the senile demented elderly: a pilot study. Gerontologist 26:158–163

Huang L, Cartwright W, Hu T (1988) The economic cost of senile dementia in the United States, 1985. Public Health Rept 103:3–7

Jorm AF, Korten AE, Henderson AS (1987) The prevalence of dementia: A quantitative integration of the literature. Acta Psych Scand 76:464–479

Jorm AF, Korten AE, Jacomb PA (1988) Projected increases in the number of dementia cases for 29 developed countries: application of a new method for making projections. Acta Psych Scand 78:493–500

Katzman R, Kawas CH (1994) The epidemiology of dementia and Alzheimer disease. In: Terry RD, Katzman R, Bick KL (eds) Alzheimer disease. Raven Press, New York, pp 105–122

Katzman R, Zhang M, Qu W-Y, Wang Z, Liu WT, Yu E, Wong S-C, Salmon D, Grant I (1988) A Chinese version of the mini-mental state examination: Impact of illiteracy in a Shanghai dementia survey. J Clin Epidemiol 41:971–978

Kokmen E, Beard CM, O'Brien PC, Kurland LT (1996) Epidemiology of dementia in Rochester, Minnesota. Mayo Clin Proc 71(3):275–282

Max W, Webber PA, Fox PJ (1995) Alzheimer's disease. The unpaid burden of caring. J Aging Health 7:179–199

McKhann G, Drachman D, Folstein M, Katzman R, Price D, Stadlan EM (1984) Clinical diagnosis of Alzheimer's disease: a report of the NINCDS-ADRDA work group under the auspices of the Department of Health and Human Services task force on Alzheimer's disease. Neurology, 34:939–944

Olichney JM, Hansen LA, Hofstetter CR, Grundman M, Katzman R, Thal LJ (1995) Cerebral infarction in Alzheimer's disease is associated with severe amyloid angiopathy and hypertension. Arch Neurol 52:702–708

Østbye T, Crosse E (1994) Net economic costs of dementia in Canada. Can Med Assoc J 151:1457–1464

Rice DR, Fox PJ, Max W (1993) The economic burden of Alzheimer's disease care. Health Affairs 12: 165–176

Rocca WA, Hofman A, Brayne C, Breteler MMB, Clarke M, Copeland JRM, Dartigues J-F, Engedal K, Hagnell O, Heeren TJ, Jonker C, Lindesay J, Lobo A, Mann AH, Mölsä PK, Morgan K, O'Connor DW, da Silva Droux A, Sulkava R, Kay DWK, Amaducci L (1991) Frequency and distribution of Alzheimer's disease in Europe: A collaborative study of 1980–1990 prevalence findings. Ann Neurol 30:381–390

Román GC, Tatemichi TK, Erkinjuntti T, Cummings JL, Masdeu JC, Garcia JH, Amaducci L, Orgogozo JM, Brun A, Hofman A, Moody DM, O'Brien MD, Yamaguchi T, Grafman J, Drayer BP, Bennet DA, Fisher M, Ogata J, Kokmen E, Bermejo F, Wolf PA, Gorelick PB, Bick KL, Pajeau AK, Bell MA, DeCarli C, Culebras A, Korczyn AD, Bogousslavsky J, Hartmann A, Scheinberg P (1993) Vascular dementia: diagnostic criteria for research studies. Report of the NINDS-AIREN International Workshop. Neurology 43:250–260

Rosen WG, Terry RD, Fuld PA, Katzman R, Peck A (1980) Pathological verification of ischemic score in differentiation of dementias. Ann Neurol 7:486–488

Shaji S, Promodu K, Abraham T, Roy KJ, Verghese A (1996) An epidemiological study of dementia in a rural community in Kerala, India. Brit J Psych 168:745–749

Souêtre EJ, Qing W, Vigoureux I, Dartigues JF, Lozet H, Lacomblez L, Derouesne C (1995) Economic analysis of Alzheimer's disease in outpatients: impact of symptom severity. Int Psychogeriatrics 7(1):115–122

Stommel M, Collins CE, Given BA (1994) the costs of family contributions to the care of persons with dementia. Gerontologist 34:199–205

Tang MX, Stern Y, Marder K, Bell K, Gurland B, Lantigua R, Andrews H, Feng L, Tycko B, Mayeux R (1998) The APOE-epsilon4 allele and the risk of Alzheimer disease among African Americans, whites, and Hispanics. JAMA 279:751–755

Ueda K, Kawano H, Hasuo Y, Fujishima M (1992) Prevalence and etiology of dementia in a Japanese community. Stroke 23:798–803

United Nations (1998) World population prospects: the 1996 revision. Population division of the Department of Economic and Social Affairs of the United Nations Secretariat, Washington, DC

US Bureau of the Census Statistical Abstract of the Unites States, 1997 (117th Edition). Washington, DC

Weinberger M, Gold DT, Divine GW, Cowper PA, Hodgson LG, Schreiner PJ, George LK (1993) Expenditures in caring for patients with dementia who live at home. Am J Public Health 83:338–341

Welch HG, Walsh JS, Larson EB (1992) The cost of institutional care in Alzheimer's disease: Nursing home and hospital use in a prospective cohort. J Am Geriatrics Soc 40:221–224

Wimo A, Karlsson G, Sandman PO, Corder L, Winblad B (1997) Cost of illness due to dementia in Sweden. Int J Geriatric Psych 12:857–861

Yoshitake T, Kiyohara Y, Kato I, Ohmura T, Iwamoto H, Nakayama K, Ohmori S, Nomiyama K, Kawano H, Ueda K (1995) Incidence and risk factors of vascular dementia and Alzheimer's disease in a defined elderly Japanese population: the Hisayama Study. Neurology 45:1161–1168

Zhang M, Katzman R, Jin H, Cai G, Wang Z, Qu G, Grant I, Yu E, Levy P, Liu WT (1990) The prevalence of dementia and Alzheimer's disease (AD) in Shanghai, China: Impact of age, gender and education. Ann Neurol 27:428–437

Predicting Who Will Develop Alzheimer's Disease

*R. Mayeux**

Introduction

Despite several decades of remarkable progress in research, Alzheimer's disease remains the most frequent cause of dementia and one of the most disabling diseases among the elderly. Traditionally, the definitive diagnosis of Alzheimer's disease has been reserved for the postmortem examination. A general loss of neurons, the deposition of β-amyloid in the form of dense plaques with neuritic elements and the presence of neurofibrillary tangles that contain intraneuronal paired helical filaments composed of an abnormally phosphorylated *tau* protein are the defining morphological characteristics of this disease. However, recently it has become evident that the clinical diagnosis is remarkably accurate (Burns et al. 1990; Wade et al. 1987; Risse et al. 1990; Gearing et al. 1995); evident that the clinical diagnosis is remarkably accurate the antemortem diagnosis is correct 90 % of the time (Mayeux et al. 1998). A decline in memory and the loss of other cognitive skills in an elderly individual without other medical or psychiatric illness usually lead to a clinical assessment in which the diagnosis of Alzheimer's disease is considered.

The preclinical or "asymptomatic" diagnosis of Alzheimer's disease is an important goal and one that is actively being researched. Brain imaging (Van Gool et al. 1995; Lavenu et al. 1997), psychological testing (Masur et al. 1994; Jacobs et al. 1995) and other (Lee et al. 1996) procedures have been used to identify individuals who either do not have symptoms or signs or have only minimal indications of Alzheimer's disease. These methods, while encouraging, may not be appropriate for use in primary or secondary prevention. Individuals with subtle brain lesions or evidence of cognitive failure may already have profound pathological changes. For primary and secondary prevention, the task of determining who will develop Alzheimer's disease before there are any clinical signs or symptoms or any indications of pathology is a daunting task, but one that is essential.

It has become clear that several genes can play a role in the etiology and pathogenesis of Alzheimer's disease. Mutations in the amyloid precursor protein (APP) and presenilin I and II (PS1, PS2) result in a dominantly inherited form of

* The Gertrude H. Sergievsky Center, 630 West 168th Street, Columbia University, New York, NY 10032. Voice: 212-305-2391, FAX: 212-305-2518, email: rpm2@columbia.edu.

R. Mayeux / Y. Christen (Eds.)
Epidemiology of Alzheimer's Disease:
From Gene to Prevention

the disease that usually begins before the age of 60 years and has been found to alter amyloid β (Aβ) protein metabolism, a major constituent of the neuritic plaque found in the brains of patients with Alzheimer's disease. Mutations in these three genes account for more than half of the patients with this form of the disease, but these early-onset familial forms probably represent less than 5 % of afflicted individuals.

Familial and sporadic forms of Alzheimer's disease occurring later in life have been associated with the ε4 polymorphism in the gene encoding apolipoprotein-E (APOE). The attributable risk for APOE-ε4 may be as high as 40 % in some populations. However, the strength of the association between APOE-ε4 and Alzheimer's disease varies with age (Evans et al. 1997a; Farrer et al. 1997), ethnic background (Maestre et al. 1995; Tang et al. 1998), heart disease (Hofman et al. 1997) and other risk factors (Mayeux et al. 1995). Nevertheless, the APOE genotype has become one of the most important determinants of Alzheimer's disease.

Other genes or even environmental factors are also likely to be related or influence the risk of developing any form of Alzheimer's disease. The risk of disease may depend on the number and impact of the contributing risk factors rather than on the presence or absence of a single polymorphism or exposure to a single risk factor. Any two individuals with different genetic backgrounds or with different environmental exposures would be expected to differ in their risk of developing Alzheimer's disease, even if they both had the same APOE genotype. In fact, as will be discussed here, other genes and risk factors that could interact with APOE-ε4 have already been identified. Nevertheless, our genetic background is established at birth long before any signs or symptoms of Alzheimer's disease have begun. It is therefore quite possible that risk assessment will depend almost entirely on a genetic analysis that includes some information regarding exposure to other factors.

Measurement of Disease Risk in Alzheimer's Disease

To establish a cause in epidemiology requires that individuals exposed to a risk factor be clearly distinguished from those not exposed. Similarly, those individuals with disease should be differentiated from those who are disease free, which is usually clear in this disease. The measurement of risk is relative, in which the probability of developing disease associated with a particular risk factor is compared to the probability of developing disease in its absence. The two frequently used measures of association forming the basis for estimating disease risk are the odds ratio and the relative risk. The odds ratio, usually calculated from cross-sectional or case-control studies, is the ratio of the odds that a case has the genetic mutation or polymorphism in question or has been exposed to a risk factor compared with the odds that a control has similar genetic background or exposure. For prospective cohort studies, where genotype and exposure information are obtained before disease occurs, the relative risk is calculated; that is, the risk of developing disease among gene carriers or those exposed to the risk among those without the gene or those unexposed. Both the odds ratio and the relative risk reflect the magnitude of the association between a disease like Alzheimer's disease and a specific mutation in a gene or an environmental factor. Risk can also be measured in terms of absolute differences, in which the rate of disease among those exposed to the risk factor is estimated by subtracting the rate of disease among those unexposed. The risk difference, or attributable risk, is not as broadly used but estimates the degree of risk related to a particular risk factor after all other factors related to the disease are considered. These related measurements that can be used to estimate the disease burden attributable to a particular factor include the calculation of attributable risk.

Evaluating the association between individual risk factors and Alzheimer's disease can be subject to several potential sources of bias. This is most evident in case-control studies in which the history of exposure is ascertained from an informant, not the patient. Bias in the recall of specific exposures and the temporal order of the association seriously limit the interpretation and usefulness of some observations. Even when the risk factor is a genetic polymorphism in a case-control study, the possibility that the association is related to survival cannot be eliminated entirely. Several major prospective studies have identified antecedent factors that may lend themselves to an accurate method for establishing who is at risk for Alzheimer's disease.

Antecedent Factors Associated with Alzheimer's Disease

Age

The proportion of individuals with Alzheimer's disease increases with each decade of life to a peak after age 80 of approximately 30 % to 40 %. Incidence rates, which reflect the number of new cases in a given time period, also follow this age-related trend, with the peak incidence of between 6 % and 8 % occurring after age 80. In East Boston, Evans et al. (1989) reported that the proportion of individuals with Alzheimer's disease, including both mild and severe forms, increases 15-fold from 3 % between the ages of 65 and 74 to 47 % for those age 85 and older. The number of new cases developing each year also rises steadily between these ages, from 0.5 % per year between ages 65 and 70 to nearly 6 % to 8 % after age 85 (Herbert et al. 1995). There are insufficient data among individuals over 85 years of age to draw specific conclusions, but the trend appears to continue (Rocca et al. 1998). While younger individuals can and do develop Alzheimer's disease, it remains a rare occurrence before the age of 50.

Some, but not all, of the pathological features of Alzheimer's disease occur in the brains of normal elderly who die without a history of dementia. However, Alzheimer's disease is clearly distinguishable from normal age-related changes, indicating that it is a specific disease process. Thus, while advancing age is strongly associated with an increased risk of developing the disease, it is not a direct cause; neither is Alzheimer's disease a consequence of the aging process.

Gender

The frequency of Alzheimer's disease may be higher among women than men (Rocca et al. 1990; Zhang et al. 1990), though not all investigations have found this trend (Fratiglioni et al. 1991; Fichter et al. 1995). In several studies the overall incidence rates for Alzheimer's disease were higher for women than men (Katzman et al. 1989; Rocca et al. 1991; Gussekloo et al. 1995). Among individuals aged 85 years or more, Gussekloo et al. (1995) found a higher risk for women than men (8.9 % vs 2.7 %), but others have not observed differences for men and women (Letenneur et al. 1994).

APOE-ε4 related risk may be higher among women than men, but this issue remains controversial. Farrer et al. (1995) found that the risk of developing Alzheimer's disease was higher among female, compared to male, relatives of patients. Devi et al. (1998) confirmed this observation among female relatives of patients who were African-Americans, Caucasians and Hispanics. Corder et al. (1995) suggested that men with Alzheimer's disease do not survive as well as women with this disease. Therefore, women appear to have a slightly higher risk of Alzheimer's disease and survive longer than men once the disease has begun. As with advancing age, gender may be indirectly associated with the cause of Alzheimer's disease but is not a direct cause.

Education and Occupation

The risk of Alzheimer's disease has been consistently observed to be higher among individuals with little or no formal education (Zhang et al. 1990; Rocca et al. 1991; Stern et al. 1994). Adjusting for age and gender, Stern et al. (1994) reported that the relative risk of developing AD was increased two-fold among those with less than eight years of education or with low occupational attainment. There have been two studies that found no difference in risk related to education. Using the record-linkage system from the Mayo Clinic in Rochester, Beard et al. (1992) found no difference between the educational level of cases with Alzheimer's disease and controls who had been matched to cases on gender, age and duration of medical record. Cobb et al. (1995), using data from the Framingham study of incident dementia and Alzheimer's disease, concluded that low educational attainment was not a risk factor. It is possible that the range of education in the Rochester cohort and that in Framingham was sufficiently homogeneous as to preclude the identification of education as a risk factor.

Education may represent a proxy for other exposures that are the actual risk factors. Individuals with less education might be exposed to unique toxic or environmental exposures or nutritional deficiencies that have not, as yet, been characterized. Evans et al. (1997b) have suggested that the process of education increases synaptic growth and thereby provides a clinical reserve against the pathological consequences of Alzheimer's disease.

Traumatic Head Injury

An association between Alzheimer's disease and prior traumatic head injury has been observed by several investigators (Mayeux et al. 1993, 1995; Canadian Study of Health and Aging 1994; Rasmusson et al. 1995; O'Meara et al. 1997). Even for studies in which the association was not statistically significant, the frequency of head injury was always increased in patients compared with controls. Because earlier studies were retrospective in design, each may have been affected by recall bias and it was impossible to establish the temporal relationship between the onset of dementia and the head injury. Two prospective cohort studies failed to find an association between Alzheimer's disease and head injury (Katzman et al. 1989; Williams et al. 1991), but Schofield et al. (1997) found that a history of head injury was associated with earlier onset of AD in a prospective cohort study. A head injury that occurred after the age of 45 years was associated with a in-fold increase in the risk of AD (Schofield et al. 1997).

An up-regulation of the amyloid precursor protein (APP) suggests increased amyloid deposition as a consequence of head injury (Roberts et al. 1994). Head injury might also cause neuronal loss that results directly in cognitive impairment or might increase susceptibility to Alzheimer's disease.

Down Syndrome

Virtually every individual with Down Syndrome living to age 40 develops the pathological changes of Alzheimer's disease in brain (Mann and Esiri 1989). Many patients with Down Syndrome, though not all, have an associated cognitive decline. Because the gene encoding APP, is located on chromosome 21, it seems very likely that the development of Alzheimer's disease in the brain of individuals with Down's syndrome is an immediate consequence of excess amyloid production, due to the trisomic gene. Aβ is a secreted peptide that yields Aβ1–40 and Aβ1–42, both of which are in varying concentrations in cerebrospinal fluid (CSF) and plasma (Scheuner et al. 1996). In familial Alzheimer's disease caused by mutations in the APP, PSI and PSII genes and in Down Syndrome, plasma levels of Aβ42 are elevated relative to controls and individuals without these gene mutations (Scheuner et al. 1996; Kosaka et al. 1997).

The risk of Alzheimer's disease associated with a family history of Down Syndrome appears to be increased two- to three-fold. Schupf et al. (1994) investigated the familial risk of Alzheimer's disease among the families of adults with Down Syndrome. Because most of the nondisjunction events in Down Syndrome are of maternal origin, they postulated that an increased frequency of Alzheimer's disease might be present among mothers but not fathers. They proposed that this shared susceptibility involves an accelerated aging process, leading to the birth of a child with Down Syndrome in relatively young mothers and to increased risk of dementia in the mother as well as her relatives. Indeed, among the family members of persons with Down Syndrome they found the risk of an

Alzheimer's disease-like dementia among mothers who were young (less than 35 years old) when their child with Down Syndrome was born was five times that of mothers who had children with other types of mental retardation, whereas the risks of dementia among mothers who were older (over age 35) at the proband's birth were comparable to those of mothers of children with other types of mental retardation.

Family History and Genetic Mutations and Polymorphisms

The risk of developing Alzheimer's disease may be increase two- to four-fold among individuals who have a first degree relative with the disease, and the risk may be even higher when two or more relatives are affected (Devi et al. 1998; van Duijn et al. 1991). While the familial occurrence of a disease may reflect non-genetic mechanisms, such as shared environmental exposures, the overwhelming consensus is that genes play a major role in the etiology of Alzheimer's disease.

Familial Alzheimer's disease, inherited in an autosomal dominant pattern, has been described in numerous families worldwide (Bird 1994). Although affected individuals from these kindreds comprise a small proportion of Alzheimer's disease overall, the studies of these families are of major importance because they provide clues to the fundamental mechanisms of the disease. As described earlier, genes on three different chromosomes have been found in families with autosomal dominant Alzheimer's disease beginning before the fifth decade of life (St Georg-Hyslop et al. 1987, 1992; Sherrington et al. 1995; Levy-Lahad et al. 1995 a, b). Mutations in the APP gene on chromosome 21 results in an overexpression of the β amyloid protein and the accumulation of amyloid deposits in brain, but how this causes Alzheimer's disease is unknown (Selkoe 1997; Hutton and Hardy 1997). The presenilin genes on chromosome 14 (PSI) and chromosome 1 (PSII) encode similar transmembrane proteins (Sherrington et al. 1995; Levy-Lahad et al. 1995 a, b; Kovacs et al. 1996) that are involved in intercellular signaling (Levitan and Greenwald 1995) and amyloid metabolism (Scheuner et al. 1996).

Phenotypes associated with each of these mutations differ in that PS1 is associated with a rapidly progressive form of the disease beginning betweeen the ages of 30 and 40 years and complete penetrance, whereas the PS2 mutation has a more variable age-at-onset with incomplete penetrance. Mutations in the APP gene have been associated with onset between the ages of 40 and 60 years of age. Age at onset within the APP families appears consistent, but can be modified by other factors such as the APOE. These three genes are considered deterministic, in that individuals with these mutations almost always develop the disease phenotype.

The pioneering work of Pericak-Vance et al. (1991) led to the eventual association between APOE-ε4 and Alzheimer's disease, now replicated in laboratories worldwide (Farrer et al. 1997; Roses 1996). The evidence supporting APOE-ε4 as a susceptibility gene has been compelling: 1) in Caucasians, APOE-ε2, and to a lesser extent ε3, reduces risk (Corder et al. 1994); 2) APOE-ε4 decreases the age-at-onset of familial AD with the APP mutation (Levy-Lahad and Bird 1996); 3) APOE-ε4 decreases the age-at-onset of dementia in Down Syndrome (Schupf et al. 1996). In familial late-onset Alzheimer's disease, each ε4 allele lowers the age-at-onset by 7 to 9 years (Corder et al. 1993). Individuals with one ε4 allele have a 25 to 40 % chance of developing Alzheimer's disease, but individuals without the ε4 allele are still at risk. The risk of Alzheimer's disease related to the APOE-ε4 allele was reported to be weaker in Hispanics, Africans and African-Americans than in Caucasians (Farrer et al. 1997; Maestre et al. 1995; Tang et al. 1998) and there was no protective effect of APOE-ε2 (Hendrie et al. 1995; Sahota et al. 1997). In the absence of an APOE-ε4 allele, the absolute risk of Alzheimer's disease is four times higher for African-Americans and three times higher for Hispanics compared with Caucasians (Tang et al. 1998). In comparison the absolute risk of Alzheimer's disease with an APOE-ε4 allele was similar across the ethnic groups.

APOE is the most upstream member of a large cluster of apolipoprotein genes that are co-regulated in some tissues by the interaction of the promoters of the individual genes with a set of shared enhancer elements (Simonet et al. 1991, 1993; Smit et al. 1988). A number of preliminary studies have shown that a sequence variant in the promoter of the APOC1 gene, located near APOE and variants in the APOE promoter regions, associates strongly with AD in Caucasian populations (Chartier-Hardlin et al. 1994; Poduslo et al. 1995; Bullido et al. 1998).

Polymorphisms in several other genes have been associated with Alzheimer's disease, though most lack independent confirmation. An intron in the PS1 gene (Wragg et al. 1996; Higuchi et al. 1996; Kehoe et al. 1996), the alpha-1 antichymotrypsin gene (Kamboh et al. 1995; Gilfix and Briones 1997; Haines et al. 1996) HLA-A2 (Payami et al. 1997) and butyrylcholinesterase (Lehmann et al. 1997) may also harbor polymorphisms altering AD risk independently or by interaction with APOE. A mutation found in 70 % of Alzheimer's disease patients in the cytochrome *c* oxidase genes in the mitochondrial genome (Davis et al. 1997) has been identified by Hirano et al. (1997) and others (Wallace et al. 1997) to be a nuclear encoded pseudogene. Polymorphisms in the gene encoding bleomycin hydroxylase on chromosome 17 have been associated with late-onset sporadic Alzheimer's disease in one study, but remains unconfirmed (Farrer et al. 1998).

Pericak-Vance et al. (1997) and Rogaeva et al. (1998) found linkage to chromosome 12 in families with Alzheimer's disease, independent of the APOE-ε4 allele. Wu et al. (1998) were unable to confirm the linkage but, using the same families, Blacker et al. (1998) reported an association with the alpha-2-macroglobulin gene on chromosome 12 near the linkage site. The genetic association to the alpha-2 macroglobulin gene has not yet been confirmed.

Risk Assessment Leads to Disease Prevention

Risk factors represent characteristics in personal behavior or lifestyle, an environmental exposure, or an inherited gene that, on the basis of epidemiologic evidence, are associated with disease. By virtue of their presence, risk factors indicate individuals who are at higher (or lower) risk of disease relative to individuals without the risk factor. Modification of these risk factors may reduce the chances of developing the disease, delay the onset of disease or prevent the disease altogether. Preventing disease by these means requires early detection by screening individuals who carry risk genes or have exposures that influence risk of disease and are asymptomatic. Unlike case finding, screening for "high risk" individuals usually involves a community or a stable, healthy population. There are minimum requirements for community-based screening programs, including the following: 1) the disease must be serious or life-threatening; 2) there must be an effective therapy; 3) the natural history must be understood; and 4) the disease must not be too rare or too common so that effective screening methods can be developed.

The possibility of using screening methods to identify individuals susceptible to Alzheimer's disease leads to a careful consideration of these requirements. The disease does shorten life span (88). While there are treatments available, none are regarded as "effective" by any means. Studies have carefully mapped the natural history of Alzheimer's disease (Piccini et al. 1995; Stern et al. 1997 a, b; Heyman et al. 1997; Thomas et al. 1997; Albert et al. 1997) and it is frequent enough to deserve our attention.

Primary and secondary prevention would involve identifying healthy men and women who are at higher than average risk of developing Alzheimer's disease. For example, individuals homozygous or heterozygous for the APOE-ε4 allele or those with a family history of Alzheimer's disease in a parent or sibling or another risk factor might be considered at "high risk." It would be reasonable to start with safe compounds with low adverse effect profiles, such as anti-inflammatory agents (Stewart et al. 1997), estrogen (Tang et al. 1996) or even anti-oxidants such as vitamin C (Paleologos et al. 1998). However, strategies for effective primary or secondary prevention are only now being developed. Nonetheless, in the future ascertainment of genetic profiles and risk assessment will most likely be used to identify individuals at risk for Alzheimer's disease.

Acknowledgments

Support was provided by Federal Grants AG07232, AG10963, AG08702, NS15076 and RR00645, The Taub Foundation, the Charles S. Robertson Memorial Gift for Alzheimer's Disease Research from the Banbury Fund and the Blachette Hooker Rockefeller Foundation.

References

Albert SM, Sano M, Marder K, Jacobs DM, Brandt J, Albert M, Stern Y (1997) Participation in clinical trials and long-term outcomes in Alzheimer's disease. Neurology (49:38–43.
Allan CM, Taylor S, Taylor JM (1997) Two hepatic enhancers, HCR. 1 and HCR. 2, coordinate liver expression of the entire human apolipoprotein E/CI/CIV/CII gene cluster. J Biol Chem. 272:29113–29119
Beard CM, Kokmen E, Offord KP, Kurland LT (1992) Lack of association between Alzheimer's disease and education, occupation, martial status, or living arrangement. Neurology 42:2063–2068
Bird TD (1994) Clinical genetics of Alzheimer's disease: In: Terry RD, Katzman R, Bick KL (eds) Alzheimer's disease. New York, Raven Press pp 65–74
Blacker, D, Wilcox MA, Laird NM, Rodes L, Horvath SM, Go RCP, Perry B, Watson B, Bassett SS, McInnis MG, Albert MS, Hyman BT, Hyman RE (1998) Alpha-2-macroglobulin is genetically associated with Alzheimer disease. Nat Genet 19:357–360
Bullido MJ, Artiga MJ, Recuero M, Sastre I, Garcia MA, Aldudo J, Lendon C, Han SW, Morris JC, Frank A, Vazquez J, Goate A, Valdivieso F (1998) A polymorphism in the regulatory region of APOE associated with risk of Alzheimer's dementia. Nature Genet 18:69–71
Burns A, Luther P, Levy R, Jacoby R, Lantos P (1990) Accuracy of clinical diagnosis of Alzheimer's disease. Brit Med J 301:1026
Canadian Study of Health and Aging (1994) The Canadian study of health and aging: risk factors for Alzheimer's disease in Canada. Neurology 44:2073–2080
Chartier-Harlin M-C, Parfitt M, Legrain S, Perez-Tur J, Brousseau T, Evans A, Berr C, Vidal O, Roques P, Gourlet V, Fruchard JC, Delacourte A, Rossor M, Amouyel P (1994) Apolipoprotein E, ε4 allele as a major risk factor for sporadic early and late-onset forms of Alzheimer's disease: analysis of the 19q13.2 chromosomal region. Hum. Mol Genet 3:569–574
Cobb JL, Wolf PA, Au R, White R, D'Agostino RB (1995). The effect of education on the incidence of dementia and Alzheimer's disease in the Framingham Study. Neurology 45:1707–1712
Corder EH, Saunders AM, Strittmatter WJ, Schmechel DE, Gaskell PC, Small GW, Roses AD, Haines JL, Pericak-Vance MA (1993) Gene dose of apolipoprotein E type 4 allele and the risk of Alzheimer's disease in late onset families. Science 261: 828–829
Corder EH, Saunders AM, Risch NJ, Strittmatter WJ, Schmechel DE, Gaskell Jr PC, Rimmler JB, Locke PA, Conneally PM, Schmader KE, Small GW, Roses AD, Haines JL, Pericak-Vance MA (1994) Protective effect of apolipoprotein E type 2 allele for late onset Alzheimer disease. Nat Genet 7:180–184
Corder EH, Saunders AM, Strittmatter WJ, Schmechel DE, Gaskell PC, Rimmler JB, Locke PA, Conneally PM, Schmader KE, Tanzi RE, Gusella JF, Small GW, Roses AD, Pericak-Vance MA, Haines JL (1995) Apolipoprotein E, survival in Alzheimer's disease patients, and the competing risks of death and Alzheimer's disease. Neurology 45: 1323–1328
Davis RE, Miller S, Herrnstadt C, Ghosh SS, Fahy E, Shinobu LA, Galaskos D, Thal LJ, Beal F, Howell N, Parker WD (1997) Mutations in mitochondrial cytochrome *c* oxidase genes segregate with late-onset Alzheimer disease. Proc Natl Acad Sci USA 94:4526–4531
Devi G, Ottman R, Tang, M-X, Marder K, Stern Y, Mayeux R (1998) Familial aggregation of Alzheimer's disease and the influence of apolipoprotein E genotype in Caucasians, African Americans and Caribbean Hispanics in Northern Manhattan, Ann Neurol 44:496
Evans DA, Funkenstein HH, Albert MS, Scherr PA, Cook NR, Chown MJ, Heber LE, Hennekens CH, Taylor JO (1989) Prevalence of Alzheimer's disease in a community population of older persons. JAMA 262:2551–2556
Evans DA, Beckett LA, Field TS, Feng L, Albert MS, Bennett DA, Tycko B, Mayeux R (1997 a) Apolipoprotein E4 and incidence of Alzheimer's disease in a community population of older persons. JAMA 277:822–824
Evans DA, Hebert LE, Beckett LA, Scherr PA, Albert MS, Chown MJ, Pilgrim DM, Taylor JO (1997 b) Education and other measures of socioeconomic status and risk of incident Alzheimer disease in a defined population of older persons. Arch Neurol 54: 1399–1405
Farrer LA, Cupples LA, van Duijn CM, Kurtz A, Zimmer R, Müller U, Green RC, Clarke V, Shoffner J, Wallace DC, Chui H, Flanagan SD, Duara R, St. George-Hyslop P, Auerbach SA, Volicer L, Wells JM,

van Broeckhoven C, Growdon JH, Haines JL (1995) Apolipoprotein E genotype in patients with Alzheimer's disease: implications for the risk of dementia among relatives. Ann Neurol 38:797–808

Farrer LA, Cupples LA, Haines JL, Hyman B, Kukull WA, Mayeux R, Myers RH, PericaKaVance MA, Risch N, van Duijn CM (1997) Effects of age, gender and ethnicity on the association between apolipoprotein-E genotype and Alzheimer's disease. JAMA 278: 1349–1356.

Farrer LA, Abraham CR, Haines JL, Rogaera EA, Song Y, McGraw WT, Brindle N, Premkumar S, Scott WK, Yamaoka LH, Saunders AM, Roses AD, Auerbach SA, Sorbi S, Duara R, Pericak-Vance MA, St. George-Hyslop PH (1998) Association between bleomyscin hydrolase and Alzheimer disease in Caucasians. Ann Neurol 44:808–811

Fichter MM, Meller I, Schröppel H, Steinkirchner R (1995) Dementia and cognitive impairment in the oldest old in the community: prevalence and comorbidity. Br J Psychiat 166:621–629

Fratiglioni L, Grut M, Forsell Y, Viitanen M, Grafstrom M, Holmen K, Ericsson K, Backmann L, Ahlbom A, Winblad B (1991) Prevalence of Alzheimer's disease and other dementias in an elderly urban population: relationship with age, sex and education. Neurology 41:1886–1892

Gearing M, Mirra SS, Hedreen JC, Sumi SM, Hansen LA, Heyman A (1995) The Consortium to Establish a Registry for Alzheimer's Disease (CERAD). Part X. Neuropathology confirmation of the clinical diagnosis of Alzheimer's disease. Neurology 45:461–466

Gilfix BM, Briones L (1997) absence of the A1252G mutation in alpha 1-antichymotrypsin in a North American population suffering from dementia. J Cereb Blood Flow Metab 17: 233–235

Gussekloo J, Heeren TJ, Izaks GJ, Ligthart GJ, Rooijmans HGM (1995) A community based study of the incidence of dementia in subjects aged 85 years and over. J Neurol Neurosurg Psychiat 59:507–510

Haines JL, Pritchard ML, Saunders AM, Schildkraut JM, Growdon JH, Gaskell PC, Farrer LA, Auerbach SA, Gusella JF, Locke PA, Rosi BL, Yamaoka L, Small GW, Conneally PM, Roses AD, Pericak-Vance M (1996) No association between alpha

Hendrie HC, Hall KS, Hui S, Unverzagt FW, Yu CE, Lahiri DK, Sahota A, Farlow M, Musick B, Class CA, Brashear A, Burdine VE, Osuntokun BO, Ogunniyi AO, Gureje O, Baiyewu O, Schellenberg GD (1995) Apolipoprotein-E genotypes and Alzheimer's disease in a community study of elderly African-Americans. Ann Neurol 37:118–120

Herbert LE, Scherr PA, Beckett LA, Albert MS, Pilgrim DM, Chown MJ, Funkenstein HH, Evans DA (1995) Age-specific incidence of Alzheimer's disease in a community population. JAMA 273:1354–1359

Heyman A, Peterson B, Fillenbaum G, Pieper C (1997) Predictors of time to institutionalization of patients with Alzheimer's disease: the CERAD experience, part XVII. Neurology 48: 1304–1309

Higuchi, S, Muramatsu T, Matsushita S, Arai H, Sasaki H (1996) Presenilin-1 polymorphism and Alzheimer's disease. Lancet 347: 1186

Hirano M, Shtilbans A, Mayeux R, Davidson MM, DiMauro S, Knowles JA, Schon EA (1997) Apparent mtDNA heteroplasmy in Alzheimer's disease patients and in normals due to PCR amplification of nucleus-embedded mtDNA pseudogenes. Proc Natl Acad Sci USA 94:14894–14899

Hofman A, Ott A, Breteler MB, Bots ML, Slooter AJ, van Harskamp F, van Duijn CN, van Broeckhoven C, Grobbee DE (1997) Atherosclerosis, apolipoprotein E, and prevalence of dementia and Alzheimer's disease in the Rotterdam Study. Lancet 349:151–154

Hutton M, Hardy M (1997) The presenilins and Alzheimer's disease. Hum Mol Genet 6:1639–1646

Jacobs DM, Sano M, Dooneief G, Marder K, Bell KL, Stern Y (1995) Neuropsychological detection and characterization of preclinical Alzheimer's disease. Neurology 45:957–962

Kamboh MI, Sanghera DK, Ferrell RE, DeKosky ST (1995) APOE*4-associated Alzheimer's disease risk is modified by alpha 1-antichymotrypsin polymorphism. Nat Genet 10: 486–488

Katzman R, Aronson M, Fuld P, Kawas C, Brown T, Morgenstern H, Frishman W, Gidez L, Eder H, Ooi WL (1989) Development of dementing illnesses in an 80-year-old volunteer cohort. Ann Neurol 25:317–324

Kehoe P, Williams J, Lovestone S, Wilcock G, Owen MJ (1996) Presenilin-1 polymorphism and Alzheimer's disease. The UK Alzheimer's Disease Collaborative Group. Lancet 347:1185

Kosaka T, Imagawa M, Seki K, Arai H, Sasaki H, Tsuji A, Asami-Odaka A, Fukushima T, Imai K, Iwatsubo T (1997) The APP717 Alzheimer mutation increases the percentage of plasma amyloid beta protein ending at A beta42(43). Neurology 48:741–745

Kovacs DM, Fausett HJ, Page KJ, Kim TW, Moir RD, Merriam DE, Hollister RD, Hallmark OG, Mancini R, Felsenstein KM, Hyman BT, Tanzi RE, Wasco W (1996) Alzheimer-associated presenilins 1 and 2: neuronal expression in brain and localization to intracellular membranes in mammalian cells. Nat Med 2:224–229

Lavenu I, Pasquier, F, Lebert F, Jacob B, Petit H (1997) Association between medial temporal lobe atrophy on CT and parietotemporal uptake decrease on SPECT in Alzheimer's disease. J Neurol Neurosurg Psychiat 63:441–445

Lee H, Swanwick GR, Coen RF, Lawlor BA (1996) Use of the clock drawing task in the diagnosis of mild and very mild Alzheimer's disease. Int Psychogeriatr 8:469–476

Lehmann DJ, Johnston C, Smith AD (1997) Synergy between the genes for butyrylcholinesterase K variant and apolipoprotein E4 in late-onset confirmed Alzheimer's disease. Hum Mol Genet 6:1933–1936

Letenneur L, Commenges D, Dartigues JF, Barberger-Gateau P, (1994) Incidence of dementia and Alzheimer's disease in elderly community residents of South-Western France. Int J Epidemiol 23:1256–1261

Levitan D, Greenwald I (1995) Facilitation of lin-12-mediated signalling by sel-12, a Caenorhabditis elegans S182 Alzheimer's disease gene. Nature 377:351–354

Levy-Lahad E, Bird TD (1996) Genetic factors in Alzheimer's disease: a review of recent advances. Ann Neurol 40:829–840

Levy-Lahad E, Wijsman EM, Nemens E, Anderson L, Goddard KA, Weber JL, Bird TD, Schellenberg GD (1995 a) A familial Alzheimer's disease locus on chromosome 1. Science 269:970–973

Levy-Lahad E, Wasco W, Poorkaj P, Romano DM, Oshima J, Pettingell WH, Yu C-E, Jondro PD, Schmidt SD, Wang K, Crowley AC, Fu Y-H, Guenette SY, Galas D, Nemens E, Wijsman EM, Bird TD, Schellenberg GD, Tanzi RE (1995 b) Candidate gene for the chromosome 1 familial Alzheimer's disease locus. Science 269:973–977

Maestre G, Ottman R, Stern Y, Gurland B, Chun M, Tang MX, Shelanski M, Tycko B, Mayeux R (1995) Apolipoprotein-E and Alzheimer's disease: ethnic variation in genotypic risks. Ann Neurol 37:254–259

Mann DMA, Esiri MM (1989) The pattern of acquisition of plaques and tangles in the brains of patients under 50 years of age with Down's syndrome J Neurol Sci 89:169–179

Masur DM, Sliwinski M, Lipton RB, Blau AD, Crystal HA (1994) Neuropsychological prediction of dementia and absence of dementia in healthy elderly persons. Neurology 44:1427–1432

Mayeux R, Ottman R, Tang MX, Noboa-Bauza L, Marder K, Gurland B, Stern Y (1993) Genetic susceptibility and Head injury as risk factors for Alzheimer's disease among community-dwelling elderly persons and their first-degree relatives. Ann Neurol 1993; 33:494–501

Mayeux R, Ottman R, Maestre G, Ngai C, Tang MX, Ginsberg H, Chun M, Tycko B, Shelanski B (1995) Synergistic effects of traumatic head injury and apolipoprotein-ε4 in patients with Alzheimer's disease. Neurology 45:555–557

Mayeux R, Saunders AM, Shea S, Mirra S, Evans D, Roses AD, Hyman BT, Crain B, Tang M-X, Phelps CH, for the Alzheimer's Disease Centers Consortium on Apolipoprotein E and Alzheimer's Disease (1998) Utility of the *APOE* genotype in the diagnosis of Alzheimer's disease. New Engl J Med 338:506–511

O'Meara ES, Kukull WA, Sheppard L, Bowen JD, McCormick WC, Teri L, Pfanschmidt M, Thompson JD, Schellenberg GD, Larson EB (1997) Head injury and risk of Alzheimer's disease by apolipoprotein E genotype. Am J Epidemiol 146:373–384

Paleologos M, Cumming RG, Lazarus R (1998) Cohort study of vitamin C intake and cognitive impairment. Am J Epidemiol 148:45–50

Payami H, Schellenberg GD, Zareparsi S, Kaye J, Sexton GJ, Head MA, Matsuyama SS, Jarvik LF, Miller B, McManus DQ, Bird TD, Katzman R, Heston L, Norman D, Small GW (1997) Evidence for association of HLA-A2 allele with onset age of Alzheimer's disease. Neurology 49:512–518

Pericak-Vance MA, Bebout JL, Gaskell Jr PC, Yamaoka LH, Hung WY, Alberts MJ, Walker AP, Bartlett RJ, Haynes CA, Welsh KA, Earl NL, Heymark A, Clark CM, Roses AD (1991) Linkage studies in familial Alzheimer disease: evidence for chromosome 19 linkage. Am J Hum Genet 48:1034–1050

Pericak-Vance MA, Bass MP, Yamaoka LH, Gaskell PC, Scott WK, Terwedow HA, Menold MM, Coneally PM, Small GW, Vance JM, Saunders AM, Roses AD, Haines JL (1997) Complete genomic screen in late-onset familial Alzheimer disease. Evidence for a new locus on chromosome 12. JAMA 278:1237–1241

Piccini C, Bracco L, Falcini M, Pracucci G, Amaducci L (1995) Natural history of Alzheimer's disease: prognostic value of plateau. J Neurol Sci 131:177–182

Poduslo SE, Neal M, Schwankhaus J (1995) A closely linked gene to apolipoprotein E may serve as an additional risk factor for Alzheimer's disease. Neurosci Lett 201:81–83

Rasmusson DX, Brandt J, Martin DB, Folstein MF (1995) Head injury as a risk factor in Alzheimer's disease. Brain Injury 9:213–219

Risse SC, Raskind MA, Nochlin D, Sumi SM, Lampe TH, Bird TD, Cubberley L, Peskind ER (1990) Neuropathological findings in patients with clinical diagnoses of probable Alzheimer's disease. Am J Psychiatry 147:168–172

Roberts GW, Gentleman SM, Lynch A, Murray L, Landon M, Graham DI (1994) β amyloid protein deposition in the brain after severe head injury: implications for the pathogenesis of Alzheimer's disease. J Neurol Neurosurg Psychiat 57:419–425

Rocca WA, Bonaiuto S, Lippi A, Luciani P, Turtu F, Cavarzeran F, Amaducci L (1990) Prevalence of clinically diagnosed Alzheimer's disease and other dementing disorders: a door-to-door survey in Appignano, Macerata Province, Italy. Neurology 40:626–631

Rocca WA, Hofman A, Brayne C, Breteler MBB, Clarke M, Copeland JRM, Dartigues J-F, Engedal K, Hagnell O, Heeren TJ, Jonker C, Lindesay J, Lobo A, Mann AH, Mölsä PK, Morgan K, O'Connor DW, da Silva Droux A, Sulkava R, Kay DWK, Amaducci L (1991) Frequency and distribution of Alzheimer's disease in Europe: a collaborative study of 1980–1990 prevalence findings. Ann Neurol 30:381–390

Rocca WA, Cha Rh, Waring SC, Kokmen E (1998) Incidence of dementia and Alzheimer's disease. Am J Epidemiol 148:51–62

Rogaeva E, Premkumar S, Song Y, Sorbi S, Brindle N, Paterson A, Duara R, Levesque G, Yu G, Nishimura M, Ikeda M, O'Toole C, Kawarai T, Jorge R, Vilarino D, Bruni AC, Farrer LA, St. George-Hyslop P (1998) Evidence for an Alzheimer disease susceptibility locus on chromosome 12 and for further locus heterogeneity. JAMA 280:614–618

Roses AD (1996) Apolipoprotein E alleles as risk factors in Alzheimer's disease. Ann Rev Med 47:387–400

Sahota A, Yang M, Gao S, Hui SL, Baiyewu O, Gureje O, Oluwole S, Ogunniyi A, Hall KS, Hendrie HC (1997) Apolipoprotein E-associated risk for Alzheimer's disease in the African-American population is genotype-dependent. Ann neurol 42:659–661

Scheuner, D, Eckman C, Jensen M, Song X, Citron M, Suzuki N, Bird TD, Hardy J, Hutton M, Kukull W, Larson E, Levy-Lahad E, Viitanen M, Peskind E, Poorkaj P, Schellenberg G, Tanzi R, Wasco W, Lannfelt L, Selkoe D, Younkin S (1996) Secreted amyloid β-protein similar to that in senile plaques of Alzheimer's disease is increased *in vivo* by the presenilin 1 and 2 and *APP* mutations linked to familial Alzheimer's disease. Nature Med 2:864–870

Schofield PW, Tang M-X, Marder K, Dooneief G, Chun M, Sano M, Stern Y, Mayeux R (1997) Alzheimer's disease after remote head injury: an incidence study. J Neurol, Neurosurg, Psychiat 62:119–124

Schupf N, Dapell D, Lee J, Ottman R, Mayeux R (1994) Increased risk for Alzheimer's disease in mothers of adults with Down syndrome. Lancet 344:353–356

Schupf N, Kapell D, Zigman W, Canto B, Tycko B, Mayeux R (1996) Onset of dementia is associated with Apolipoprotein ε4 in Down syndrome. Ann Neurol 40:799–801

Selkoe DJ (1997) Alzheimer's disease: genotypes, phenotype and treatments. Science 275:630–631

Sherrington R, Rogaev EI, Liang Y, Rogaeva EA, Levesque G, Ikeda M, Chi H, Lin C, Li G, Holman K, Tsuda T, Mar L, Foncin J-F, Bruni AC, Montessi MP, Sorbi S, Rainero I, Pinessi L, Nee L, Chumakov I, Pollen D, Brookes A, Sanseau P, Polinsky RJ, Wasco W, Da Silva HAR, Haines JL, Pericak-Vance MA, Tanzi RE, Roses AD, Fraser PE, Rommens JM, St. George-Hyslop P (1995) Cloning of a gene bearing missense mutations in early-onset familial Alzheimer's disease. Nature 375:754–760

Simonet WS, Bucay N, Pitas RE, Lauer SJ, Taylor JM (1991) Multiple tissue-specific elements control the apolipoprotein E/CI gene locus in transgenic mice. J Biol Chem 266:8651–8654

Simonet WS, Bucay N, Lauer SJ, Taylor JM (1993) A far-downstream hepatocyte-specific control region directs expression of the linked human apolipoprotein E and C-I genes in transgenic mice. J Biol Chem. 268:8221–8229

Smit M, Kooij-Meijs E, Woudt LP, Havekes LM, Frants RR (1988) Exact localization of the familial dysbetalipoproteinemia associated HpaI restriction site in the promoter region of the APOCI gene. Biochem Biophys Res Comm 152:1282–1288

Stern Y, Gurland B, Tatemichi T, Tang M, Wilder D, Mayeux R (1994) Influence of education and occupation on the incidence of Alzheimer's disease. JAMA 271:1004–1010

Stern Y, Tang MX, Albert MS, Brandt J, Jacobs DM, Bell K, Marder K, Sano M, Devanand D, Albert SM, Bylsma F, Tsai WY (1997 a) Predicting time to nursing home care and death in individuals with Alzheimer disease. JAMA 277:806–812

Stern Y, Brandt J, Albert M, Jacobs DM, Liu X, Bell K, Marder K, Sano M, Albert S, Del-Castillo Castenada C, Bylsma F, Tycko B, Mayeux R (1997 b) The absence of an apolipoprotein epsilon4 allele is associated with a more aggressive form of Alzheimer's disease. Ann Neurol 41:615–620

Stewart W, Kawas C, Corrada M, Metter E (1997) The risk of Alzheimer's disease and duration of NSAID use. Neurology 48:626–632

St George-Hyslop P, Tanzi RE, Polinsky RJ, Haines JL, Nee L, Watkins PC, Myers RH, Feldmann RG, Pollen D, Drachman D, Growdon J, Bruni A, Foncin J-F, Salmon D, Frommelt P, Amaducci L, Sorbi S, Piacentini S, Stewart GD, Hobbs WJ, Conneally PM, Gusella JF (1987) The genetic defect causing familial Alzheimer's disease maps on chromosome 21. Science 235:885–890

St George-Hyslop I, Haines J, Rogaev E, Mortilla M, Vaula G, Pericak-Vance M, Foncin J-F, Montesi M, Bruni A, Sorbi S, Rainero I, Pinessi L, Pollen D, Polinsky R, Nee L, Kennedy J, Macciardi F, Rogaeva E, Liang Y, Alexandrova N, Lukiw W, Schlumpf K, Tanzi R, Tsuda T, Farrer L, Cantu J-M, Duara R, Amaducci L, Bergamini L, Gusella J, Roses AD, Crapper McLachlan D (1992) Genetic evidence for a novel familial Alzheimer's disease locus on chromosome 14. Nature Genet 2:330–334

Tang M-X, Jacobs D, Stern Y, Marder K, Schofield P, Gurland B, Andrews H, Mayeux R (1996) Effect of oestrogen during menopause on risk and age-at-onset of Alzheimer's disease. Lancet 348:429–432

Tang M-X, Stern Y, Marder K, Bell K, Gurland B, Lantigua R, Andrews H, Feng L, Tycko B, Mayeux R (1998) APOE risks and the frequency of Alzheimer's disease among African-Americans, Caucasians and Hispanics. JAMA 279:751–755

Thomas BM, McGonigal G, McQuade CA, Starr JM, Whalley LJ (1997) Survival in early onset dementia: effects of urbanization and socio-economic deprivation. Neuroepidemiology 16:134–140

van Duijn CM, Clayton D, Chandra V, Fratiglioni L, Graves AB, Heyman A, Jorn AF, Kokmen E, Kondo K, Mortimer JA, Rocca WA, Shalat SL, Soininen H, Hofman AF (1991) Familial aggregation of Alzheimer's disease and related disorders: a collaborative reanalysis of case-control studies. Int J Epidemiol 20 (suppl 2):S 13–20

Van Gool WA, Walstra GJ, Teunisse S, Van der Zant FM, Weinstein HC, Van Royen EA (1995) Diagnosing Alzheimer's disease in elderly, mildly demented patients: the impact of routine single photon emission computed tomography. J Neurol 242:401–405

Wade JPH, Miresen TR, Hachinski VC, Fisman M, Lau C, Merskey H (1987) The clinical diagnosis of Alzheimer's disease. Arch Neurol 44:24–29

Wallace DC, Stugard C, Murdock D, Schurr T, Brown MD (1997) Ancient mtDNA sequences in the human nuclear genome: a potential source of errors in identifying pathogenic mutations. Proc Natl Acad Sci USA 94:14900–14905

Williams DB, Annegers JF, Kokmen E, O'Brien PC, Kurland LT (1991) Brain injury and neurologic sequelae: a cohort study of dementia, parkinsonism, and amyotrophic lateral sclerosis. Neurology 41:1554–1557

Wragg M, Hutton M, Talbot C (1996) Genetic association between intronic polymorphism in presenilin-1 gene and late-onset Alzheimer's disease. Alzheimer's Disease Collaborative Group. Lancet 347:509–512

Wu WS, Holmans P, Wavrant-De Vrièze F, Shears S, Kehoe P, Crook R, Booth J, Williams N, Pérez-Tur J, Roehl K, Fenton I, Chartier-Harlin M-C, Lovestone S, Williams J, Hutton M, Hardy J, Owen MJ, Goate A (1998) Genetic studies on chromosome 12 in late onset Alzheimer disease 280:619–622

Zhang MY, Katzman R, Salmon D, Jun H, Cai G, Wang Z, Qu G, Grant I, Yu E, Levy P, Klauber MR, Liu WT (1990) The prevalence of dementia and Alzheimer's disease (AD) in Shanghai, China: impact of age, gender and education. Ann Neurol 27:428–437

Genetic Factors in Early- and Late-Onset Alzheimer's Disease

*J. Tol, A. J. C. Slooter, C. M. van Duijn**

Summary

In recent years, considerable progress has been made in unravelling the genetic etiology of Alzheimer's disease (AD). Three genes have been identified that are involved in the autosomal dominant forms of early-onset AD: the β-amyloid precursor protein gene (APP) and two homologous genes, presenilin 1 (PS-1) and presenilin 2 (PS-2). Mutations in each of these genes have been found to be rare. Screening a population-based sample of patients with early-onset AD (< 65 years) revealed APP mutations in 0.5 % of the patients, PS-1 mutations in 6 % and PS-2 mutations in 1 %. Although the risk of AD for carriers of mutations in these genes is extremely high, the relative contribution of these genes to the occurrence of disease in the general population is lower than 1 %. On the population level, the apolipoprotein E (APOE) gene is a more important genetic determinant for early-onset AD as well as for the predominant, late-onset form (90–95 % of the patients). The APOE4 allele may explain up to 17 % of AD in the general population. A key issue to resolve from a public health point of view will be the interaction of this gene with drugs and other genetic and non-genetic risk factors. Large scale, long-term follow-up studies, ongoing at present, may clarify this issue. Another issue to be resolved in AD research will be the identification of other, yet unknown genes involved in the etiology of AD.

Introduction

AD is a common cause of morbidity and mortality in the elderly (Van Duijn 1996). Clinically, AD is characterized by a progressive decline in intellectual functions. The pathological characteristics of AD include the presence of β-amyloid in senile plaques and cerebral blood vessel walls and neurofibrillary tangles. Further, there are pronounced neurochemical deficits of the cholinergic, serotoninergic and monoaminergic system. It has been long recognized that genetic factors play a major role in AD (Slooter and Van Duijn 1998). In the past decades,

* Department of Epidemiology & Biostatistics Erasmus University Medical School PO BOX 1738, 3000 DR Rotterdam The Netherlands. Telephone: (+)31-10-4087394, Fax: (+)31-10-4366139, e-mail: vanduijn@epib.fgg.eur.nl.

R. Mayeux / Y. Christen (Eds.)
Epidemiology of Alzheimer's Disease:
From Gene to Prevention

important progress has been made in unraveling the genetic etiology of AD. Multiple genes have been implicated in the pathogenesis of AD (Slooter and Van Duijn 1998; Van Broeckhoven 1995; Cruts et al. 1998). In this paper, we aim to review the contribution of genetic factors to the prevalence and incidence of the disease in the general population.

Methods

To quantify the role of genetic factors in the etiology of AD, epidemiological data on family history from epidemiological studies were used. Data on family history were derived from a meta-analysis of seven population-based case-control studies (Van Duijn et al. 1991). This study comprised a total of 814 AD cases and 894 controls. Although various genes have been associated with AD, findings have been consistent for four genes (Slooter and Van Duijn 1998). In the relatively rare early-onset dominant forms, several autosomal dominant genes play a role. These include the amyloid precursor gene (APP) and the presenilin genes 1 (PS-1) and 2 (PS-2) (Slooter and Van Duijn 1998; Van Broeckhoven 1995; Cruts et al. 1998). No meta-analysis or pooled data set is available for any of the dominant genes. To estimate the contribution of these genes to AD, we used a Dutch population-based sample of presenile AD cases (age of onset <65 years; age at diagnosis <70 years). This study involved 100 cases and 118 controls (Cruts et al. 1998). The apolipoprotein E gene (APOE) (Slooter and Van Duijn 1998) has been implicated in both the early- and late-onset forms of AD. The analysis of the APOE gene is also based on a large meta-analysis of 47 studies including 5930 cases and 8607 controls (Farrer et al. 1997). Further data on the APOE genotype in incident AD cases are obtained from a large population-based study conducted in the Netherlands (Slooter et al. 1998).

AD is a multifactorial disease in which several genetic and environmental factors have been implicated. An individual may develop the disease through several pathways. Attributive risks of the exposed were calculated from the odds ratios (Hennekens and Buring 1987). The attributable risk can be interpreted as the proportion of patients that carry a genetic factor (mutation/polymorphism) in whom the disease could have been prevented by blocking the adverse effect (Rothman 1986; Hennekens and Buring 1987). To calculate the effect of the exposure to a disease in the total study population, we estimated the population attributable risk as described by Rothman (Rothman 1986). The population attributable risk will yield an estimate of the contribution of the genetic factor to the occurence of the disease in a mixed population of genetically susceptible and non-susceptible subjects.

Family History

In Table 1, risk estimates are given for family history in first degree relatives (Van Duijn et al. 1991). In patients with a relatively early onset of AD (onset before the age of 70 years), familial factors may explain 75–81 % of the disease in the exposed, that is in those with a positive family history. In cases with a positive family history the disease may be attributed to familial factors (genetic or non-genetic) in 75–81 %. At the level of the general population, 27–34 % of early-onset AD may be explained by familial factors. In patients with late-onset AD (onset after the age of 70 years), 57–62 % of the AD cases in the group of individuals with a positive family history may be attributable to familial factors. At the level of the general population, 21 % of AD may be explained by familial factors. If we compare the attributable risks of early-onset and late-onset patients, the influence of familial factors in early-onset AD is more pronounced than in late-onset AD patients. Yet the contribution of genetic factors is also expected to be considerable in patients with a late onset of disease.

Table 1. Family history of dementia in relation to the prevalence of AD in population-based studies, stratified according to age. (Van Duijn et al. 1991)

Age (years)	Proportion of exposed in the cases (%)	Odds ratio	Attributable risk (%)	Population attributable risk (%)
≤ 59	35.7	4.0	75.0	26.8
60–69	41.5	5.3	81.0	33.6
70–79	36.7	2.3	56.5	20.7
80+	33.6	2.6	61.5	20.7

Dominant genes

Table 2 provides the frequencies of the autosomal dominant AD genes in a population-based sample of early-onset AD patients in the Netherlands (Cruts et al. 1998). Although the frequency of the mutations is low among cases, frequencies in the controls are approaching 0. The latter finding may be explained in

Table 2. Contribution of autosomal dominant mutations in a population-based series of patients with early-onset AD. (Cruts et al. 1998)

Dominant genes	Proportion of exposed in the cases (%)	Odds ratio	Attributable risk (%)	Population attributable risk (%)
APP	0.5	$\propto$	≈ 100	0.5
PS1	6.0	$\propto$	≈ 100	6.0
PS2	1.0	$\propto$	≈ 100	1.0

large part by the high risk of AD in carriers. This results in odds ratios that are infinitive and attributable risks of this early-onset form of AD that approach 100 %. Thus, in all cases with a dominant mutation and an early onset of AD, the disease may be attributed to the mutation. It can be shown that, for these high risk mutations, the frequencies in patients will equal the population attributable risk. Mutations in PS-1 are by far most frequent. At the level of the general population, 6 % of AD in early-onset cases may be explained by PS-1. PS-2 and APP mutations are far more rare. Mutations in PS-2 are expected to explain 1 % of early-onset AD, APP up to 0.5 %. Although no population-based data are available on the presence of PS1, PS2 and APP in late-onset AD patients, we have estimated the contribution of PS-1, PS-2, and APP to the prevalence of disease in the general population. The rationale of the extrapolation is that all carriers of each of the dominant genes are likely to show symptoms before the age of 65 (Cruts et al. 1998). Based on population-based surveys on dementia, we assume that early-onset AD constitutes less than 1 % of the total group of AD patients. It follows from this that the three dominant genes do not explain more than 0.075 % of the occurrence of all AD.

APOE

In 3s 3 and 4, population data are given for APOE. APOE3/3 carriers are considered as a reference group. Although the odds ratio is moderately increased for heterozygotes, heterozygosity of the APOE4 allele may explain up to 17 % of the

Table 3. Contribution of the apolipoprotein E gene to the prevalence of AD in Caucasian patients (population-based). (Farrer et al. 1997)

APOE genotype	Proportion of exposed in the cases (%)	Odds ratio	Attributable risk (%)	Population attributable risk (%)
2/4	2.6	2.6	61.5	1.60
3/4	21.3	3.2	68.8	14.7
4/4	1.8	14.9	93.3	1.68
3/3	60.9	1.0		

Table 4. Apolipoprotein E and AD in a population-based series of incident patients from the Rotterdam Study. (Slooter et al. 1998)

APOE genotype	Proportion of exposed in the cases (%)	Odds ratio	Attributable risk (%)	Population attributable risk (%)
2/4	2.6	1.3	23.1	0.60
3/4	21.3	1.8	44.4	9.45
4/4	1.8	6.2	83.9	1.51
3/3	60.9	1.0		

disease in the general population, based on the data of the APOE meta-analysis (Table 3) (Farrer et al. 1997). Despite the fact that APOE4 homozygotes have a large increase in risk compared to the general population, the contribution to AD in the general population is limited (< 2 %) because of the low prevalence of this genotype. Despite the overwhelming number of studies suggesting an association between APOE4 and AD, a limited number of studies were of sufficient size to address age- and sex-specific risks. For APOE3/4 carriers, the most common AD-associated APOE genotype in cases, there is some evidence for age- and sex-specific effects in the meta-analysis by Farrer et al. (1997). The odds ratio for APOE3/4 was found to be highest at age 65 years in women (OR = 4). For men, there was no convincing evidence for age- and sex-specific APOE3/4 effects.

A concern in the studies of APOE4 in prevalent AD cases is the fact that APOE4 may be related to survival of AD. Indeed, odds ratios derived from the Rotterdam Study were found to be lower in incident AD patients (see Table 4). Based on the incident cases, up to 12 % of AD in the general population may be explained by APOE4 (Slooter et al. 1998). However, the mean age at onset of the incident patients was high, 82 years (SD 70 years). It cannot be excluded that effects are more pronounced at a younger age.

Discussion

In recent years, remarkable progress has been made in the unraveling of the genetic basis of AD. Genetic research has made a significant contribution to the understanding of the molecular etiology of the disease. Various mutations in three genes (APP, PS-1 and PS-2) have been identified which can lead to early-onset AD in particular. The three proteins causally related to AD have been identified as the β amyloid, presenilin 1 and 2 proteins. However, from a population perspective the frequency of mutations at these genes appears to be rare and limited to autosomal dominant forms of early-onset AD patients. As shown in this paper, there is a negligible proportion of AD in the population that can be attributed to these dominant mutations. The APOE4 allele is the only common genetic risk factor to date that has been consistently associated with AD in numerous studies. The risk of AD associated with this allele is more moderately increased, but because of the high frequency of this allele in the population, a larger proportion of AD may be explained by APOE4. Because of its association with the most prevalent late-onset form of AD, the APOE4 allele may explain up to 17 % of all disease in the population.

It is clear that other, yet unknown genes must be involved in the etiology of AD. Genomic searches based on classical linkage studies in extended families that are multiply affected with AD or in affected sib-pairs have not yielded reproducible results. There are several problems in the interpretation of these findings. The power of the family and sib-pair studies has been low, resulting in false negative or inconclusive findings. Part of the explanation of the negative findings may be that the disease may often result from an interplay of different genetic and environmental risk factors (Van Duijn 1996; Slooter and Van Duijn 1998). To localize such genes, which by themselves may convey only a moderate increase in risk of AD, will be difficult. There is a growing interest in the possibility of mapping disease genes through association studies using population-based patient series rather than families (Lander and Schork 1994). The statistical power of association studies is high to address candidate genes, i.e., genes that are expected to be involved in the disease. However, the chances of success are limited at present for genomic screening for yet unknown genes. For genomic searches, the situation may be more favorable in isolated populations (Lander and Schork 1994).

Ultimately, the understanding of the role of genetic factors in the risk of AD may lead to models for the disease that can be used for development of therapeutical strategies. Despite the breakthroughs in genetic research in AD, the clinical implications until now have been limited. Clinical counselling for family planning and risk prediction in asymptomatic carriers are possible for a limited number of families. However, in the absence of effective therapy or preventive strategies, the testing of asymptomatic carriers has only been performed on a limited scale. Unravelling interactions of (susceptibility) genes with preventive/risk factors may enable targeted preventive strategies. However, these studies require detailed information about genetic and non-genetic risk factors of AD from large populations. Large scale, long-term follow-up studies, ongoing at present, may further clarify the interaction between genetic and environmental factors in AD.

Acknowledgments

This paper was made possible by grants from the Netherlands Organisation for Scientific Research (NWO) and the Netherlands Institute of Health Sciences (NIHES).

References

Van Duijn CM (1996) Epidemiology of the dementias: recent developments and new approaches. JNNP 60:478–488

Slooter AJS, Van Duijn CM (1998) Genetic epidemiology of Alzheimer's disease. Epidemiol Rev 19:107–119

Van Broeckhoven C (1995) Molecular genetics of Alzheimer's disease: Identification of genes and gene mutations. Eur Neurol 35:8–19

Cruts M, Van Duijn CM, Backhovens H, Van den Broeck M, Wehnert A, Serneel S, Sherrington R, Hutton M, Hardy J, St. George-Hyslop PH Hoffmann A, van Broeckhoven C (1998) Estimation of the genetic contribution of presenilin-1 and -2 mutations in a population-based study of early-onset Alzheimer's disease. Human Molec Genet 7:43–51.

Farrer LA, Cupples LA, Haines JL, Hyman B, Kukull WA, Mayeux R, Myers RH, Pericak-Vance MA, Rish N, van Duijn CM (1997) Effects of age, sex, and ethnicity on the association between apolipoprotein E genotype and Alzheimer's disease. JAMA 278:1349–1356

Slooter AJC, Cruts M, Kalmijn S, Hofman A, Breteler MMB, Van Broeckhoven C, Van Duijn CM (1998) Apolipoprotein E and dementia. Risk estimates from a population-based incidence study: the Rotterdam Study. Arch Neurol 55 (7):964–968

Van Duijn CM, Clayton D, Chandra V, Fratiglioni L, Graves AB, Heyman A, Jorn AF, Kokmen E, Kondo K, Mortimer JA, Rocca WA, Shalat SL, Soininen H, Hofman AF (1991) Familial aggregation of Alzheimer's disease and related disorders: a collaborative re-analysis of case-control studies. Int J Epidemiol 20:S13–S20

Rothman KJ (1986) Modern epidemiology. Boston/Toronto, Little, Brown and Company

Hennekens CH, Buring JE (1987) Epidemiology in medicine. Boston/Toronto, Little, Brown and Company

Lander ES, Schork NJ (1994) Genetic dissection of complex traits. Science 265:2037–2048

Heterogeneity in Alzheimer's Disease: Implications for Epidemiology

T. S. Radebaugh, M. Ganguli**, and Z. S. Khachaturian**

Summary

It is well established that Alzheimer's is a heterogeneous disease. The heterogeneity in the disease is expressed in several domains, such as the types and patterns of clinical symptoms, the genetic underpinnings, neuropathological indices, and responses to pharmacological treatments and interventions. Much of the information published on Alzheimer's disease has been developed from highly selected patient groups. In the U.S., these patient groups are often Caucasian, middle class research volunteers. These patient groups do not represent the population of the country or the universe of people with Alzheimer's disease, and therefore there are important potential limits to the generalizability of the findings obtained. The demographic changes that are already underway, and will accelerate in the next decades in many countries in the world, will add new dimensions to the heterogeneity of the disease. Ultimately, to understand and to defeat the disease, we must understand the new cohorts of people with the disease, their genetic, environmental and social characteristics and the interactions of those characteristics. Furthermore, if we are to enlist participants in research and develop educational programs and useful and used services, then it is necessary to address a long list of social and behavioral research questions. These questions will have to be investigated against the backdrop of the anticipated changes in the demographic and cultural profiles of the people with the disease. One drug treatment, one behavioral approach, or one model for service programs will not be adequate to address the needs of all people with Alzheimer's disease. It is clear that a single size will not fit all.

Background

The results of recent epidemiological studies, or basic science discoveries bolstered and extended by epidemiological research, have had a profound impact on thinking about Alzheimer's disease. Three illustrations are: 1) the discovery that ApoE 4 is a susceptibility gene for Alzheimer's disease, 2) the national public

* Alzheimer's Association, Ronald & Nancy Reagan Research Institute, Chicago, Illinois, USA.
** University of Pittsburgh, Pittsburgh, Pennsylvania, USA.

R. Mayeux / Y. Christen (Eds.)
Epidemiology of Alzheimer's Disease:
From Gene to Prevention

health problem estimated from the prevalence data of East Boston, and 3) the emerging data indicating the differential distribution of Alzheimer's disease by ethnicity. Although epidemiological data have contributed significantly to the understanding of the disease, there are certain limitations to the generalizability of the data to other heterogeneous populations.

The vast majority of the clinical, social and behavioral information on Alzheimer's disease in the U.S. has been derived from highly selected and motivated, predominantly Caucasian, research volunteers collected in sophisticated tertiary research centers. The patient research groups do not usually represent any population. The goal has frequently been to study Alzheimer's disease in the most "pure" state, uncontaminated by other comorbid conditions, medication use, etc. This may, in some instances, be a desirable research goal. However, it may provide a skewed view and understanding of the disease as the findings are not referable to the population at large.

Recent advances lead investigators to appreciate that an avenue to understanding the biological heterogeneity of the disease at the cellular and genetic levels must begin with a more refined investigation and analysis of the people with Alzheimer's disease. Examination of people with Alzheimer's disease, their racial and ethnic backgrounds, co-morbid conditions, and circumstances leading to various exposures and experiences may provide additional clues to the nature of and origins of the disease.

Alzheimer's disease is heterogeneous, in terms of its clinical profile and comorbidities, the genetic determinants and perhaps risk factors, the social implications and consequences, and treatment responses and in the caregiving burden and societal responses. It is accepted by many that there are neuropathological variants. It may ultimately be determined that Alzheimer's disease is a group of disorders, or a final common pathway for many different pathological processes. It is important to recognize and deal with this fact in research as well as in practice and policy development. For if we extend studies from tertiary medical centers and universities into diverse populations, maintaining restrictive definitions and failing to grasp the implications of the heterogeneity of the study populations, we may not be able to systematically study the possible hypothesized variants. For example, if people with histories of alcoholism are eliminated from participation in research on Alzheimer's disease, it will never be known whether alcoholism leads to its own unique kind of non-Alzheimer's dementia or whether it is a risk factor or risk modifier for Alzheimer's disease. The same point can be expanded to include thyroid disorder, B12 deficiency, and so on.

At the moment, there is not a good way of categorizing apparent mixed dementias (the NINDS-ADRDA category of "possible Alzheimer's disease" operationally includes both uncertain and mixed cases). Therefore, the diagnostic categories, by definition, have prevented the investigation of the role and impact of comorbid conditions. It must be recognized that most people with Alzheimer's disease in the community or in institutions have important concomitant illnesses that may also impact their mental functioning. The stringency of diagnostic categories, the removal of patients from analyses because of comorbid conditions, the exclusion/inclusion criteria for entrance into investigations, and the low autopsy rate at many research sites may also be confounding the picture of the disease.

In addition to considering the more widely discussed scientific and clinical issues in the heterogeneity of Alzheimer's disease, the dimensions of heterogeneity are being expanded by population changes. It is important that investigators plan for the demographic changes and understand their implications as these changes will further complicate how we view the disease and care for people.

Demographic Changes

Many countries are undergoing profound changes in their population structures. The U.S. is experiencing a huge wave of immigration coupled with changing birthrates for population groups who are already resident. The U.S. Bureau of the Census has published massive amounts of data on the current population as well as projections for the future, much of which can be accessed through the website (http://www.census.gov). The following list, which presents a few bits of summary data and projections from the U.S. Bureau of the Census, is illustrative and was extracted from the website:

- Nearly one in ten people in U.S. is foreign born. (April 9, 1998, announcement of report "The Foreign-Born Population in the United States: March 1997" (Update))
- The U.S. is in the midst of a huge immigration wave, including a highly educated group and a poorly educated group. (April 9, 1998, announcement of report "The Foreign-Born Population in the United States: March 1997" (Update)).
- By 2050, Hispanics will be the largest minority group in the U.S., surpassing African Americans. And by 2050, Non-Hispanic Whites will make up only slightly more than 50 % of the total population.
- Many states will be non-majority states. They will be so ethnically diverse that there will be no majority group.
- In 1993, only 22 % of the U.S. population over age 25 had completed college.
- Worldwide, in both developed and developing countries, persons 65 and older are the fastest growing population group. (October 9, 1996, announcement of report "World Population Profile: 1996")
- By 2050, there will be 80 million people over the age of 65 in the U.S.
- The number of women 60 years and over worldwide is expected to more than double by 2025. (April 14, 1998, announcement of brief "Gender and Aging: Demographic Dimension").

Why should investigators in Alzheimer's disease be cognizant of the current and projected changes in the populations that they study? The answer is: as the people with the disease begin to change, it may affect what research should be done, how that research is conducted and interpreted and how the disease is understood. Simply, as the numbers of and social and cultural characteristics of populations change, there may be corresponding changes in how research should be structured. The accuracy and nature of the individual projections are less important than understanding that the changes ahead in the people with Alzheimer's disease in our clinics and service programs will add other dimensions of disease heterogeneity.

The projected demographic shifts *may* have important implications for the distribution of genetic risk factors in the upcoming generations of potential victims of Alzheimer's disease. It will be necessary to carefully examine the genetic heritage of the people from whom samples are obtained for molecular biological and molecular genetic research and to understand the distribution of purported genetic risk factors in clearly delineated population groups to which sampled material may be referred.

Although environmental risk factors are of much interest in epidemiological research, the area has proved very troublesome to investigators. One could hypothesize that the exposure to environmental and other risk factors, i.e., education, head injury, environmental pollutants, is likely to change in significant ways as the populations change. Simply, the exposure experience of the upcoming cohorts is likely to be very different from the current and previous cohorts of demented older people.

The distribution of the cultural groups will not be uniform, but some project, on the basis of current trends, that the U.S. as a whole will be increasingly segregated into enclaves of people of similar backgrounds, history and expectations. Each of the groups will bring unique genetic and exposure profiles to the table which may impact how and when the disease is expressed, resulting in varying prevalence and incidence rates and contributions of risk factors.

It is possible that the U.S. will also experience changes in the family and caregiving social structures in the upcoming decades. The dozens of significant ethnic and cultural groups hold values, religions, philosophies and expectations that will affect how services, treatment and care for demented people have to be provided to be compatible and culturally acceptable.

To engage participants in research (particularly long-term treatment or prevention trials), to effectively transmit information and educational materials about the disease, and to provide culturally compatible and helpful services, it will be necessary to have a much better understanding of who the people are and how their genetic makeup combines with their social and experiential pedigrees.

Behavioral and Social Issues

Reducing the duration of disability and shortening the period of dependency is the mission of the Alzheimer's Association scientific program, the Ronald & Nancy Reagan Research Institute. Therefore, the Behavioral and Social Research Agenda Steering Committee was established to provide advice to the Alzheimer's Association and to the scientific community on the important scientific questions in the social and behavioral arenas in Alzheimer's disease. The goal is to obtain research data that will help to *maximize functioning* including the restoration or rehabilitation of lost abilities, *prolong independence* and *maintain, or improve, the quality of life* for as long as possible for the person with Alzheimer's disease, while *minimizing familial and economic costs.* It was clearly recognized from the outset that the universe of researchable questions was enormous, so the task was to consider the questions of most importance and immediate consequence to the well being of people with the disease, their families and caregivers.

The Steering Committee is chaired by Dr. Leonard Pearlin (University of Maryland), and its members are Dr. Charlene Harrington (Univesity of California, San Francisco), Dr. Powell Lawton (Philadelphia Geriatric Center), Dr. Rhonda Montgomery (University of Kansas), and Dr. Steven Zarit (Pennsylvania State University). The Steering Committee was convened in December 1997, and its work has already helped to shape and to form the fiscal year 1999 Program Announcement of the Alzheimer's Association. The Program Announcement describes the grants program and is structured around the scientific theme of "Interventions" for Alzheimer's Disease."

The perspectives and methodologies of epidemiology coupled with the behavioral and social sciences are particularly important to the next generation of questions concerning Alzheimer's disease. This era will require a sophisticated marriage of demography and population-based field studies with much more precisely defined questions about the disease, the effectiveness of interventions and health services research. These data will in turn support the establishment of better services and programs and the application of effective preventive measures in the decades to come.

During the last few years, research on the behavioral, social, clinical and environmental aspects of Alzheimer's disease has been making impressive progress.[1] Further advances will help enhance some of the now available practical interventions, providing families with help they so desperately need. Because so little was understood, early research in the social and behavioral aspects of Alzheimer's disease focused on general questions, such as: What happened to patients and families? What were the stresses? What were the burdens? Who were the caregivers and what happened to them? Some of the early work demonstrated that Alzheimer's disease is heterogeneous. It is now well accepted that the heterogeneity characterizes not only people who suffer from the disease, but their families as well.

Research aimed at understanding the diversity, complexity and consequences of caregiving within a cultural and ethnic context, the precise nature of the problems confronting caregivers through the course of the disease, and the types and nature of effective interventions is of great importance. It has been clearly established and widely accepted that the consequences of the disease are difficult,

[1] The following discussion of behavioral and social research issues is directly extracted from the 1999 Program Announcement of the Alzheimer's Association, which can be found on the website: www.alz.org. It is presented here again to help engage epidemiologists in these questions.

but vary by social and structural and environmental characteristics. Investigators have moved beyond the establishment of and general characterization of care and management issues to a more refined dissection of the circumstances and reverberations leading to requirements for care and management. The goal is to provide carefully delineated targets and timetables for interventions and for the development of interventions and supportive services that will maintain persons with Alzheimer's disease and their families in dignity and independence for as long as possible.

In view of the enormity of the fiscal and personal problems presented by the problems occurring during the course of Alzheimer's disease, research efforts and clinical trials should be clearly targeted. Some of the most difficult symptoms include wandering, aggression, agitation, incontinence and sleep disruption. The long-term goal is to understand the neurobiological basis of these symptoms. The more immediate goal is to interrupt or prevent behavioral symptoms so that the person with Alzheimer's disease and the family are not so battered, to enhance functioning and independence of the person with Alzheimer's disease, and to improve the quality of life for the person with Alzheimer's disease, the family and caregivers.

Examples of questions that illustrate research needs are presented below. Each question must be posed and studied in a manner that will address the demographic changes underway. The answers must be relevant to all groups of people in need.

- Evaluation research aimed at determining effectiveness, including cost effectivenesses, of practical programs already underway. Chapters of the Alzheimer's Association, and other organizations, have been very creative in developing practical programs, but evaluation of the outcomes has been lacking. There has been no mechanism for finding out what works (or does not), under what circumstances, for *whom* and why.
- The use of personal care and attendant services in the home has been growing. Scant research data exist on these services, the outcomes for the person with Alzheimer's disease, cost effectiveness, and conditions under which the services are most useful and acceptable. How do the cultural and other social characteristics of the person with Alzheimer's disease and the family influence the use and acceptability of these services?
- Interventions aimed at preventing, interrupting or reducing specific behavioral difficulties (i.e., aggression, wandering, urinary incontinence) associated with the progression of Alzheimer's disease are of particular importance. These interventions must be socially and cultural appropriate.
- There has been substantial research on family caregiving, but many subgroups of people with Alzheimer's disease have received little research attention. More information is required on the problems of low income people, particularly those who are living alone or who are homeless, and cultural and ethnic minority groups. What happens to them, what are their needs, how can these needs be met most effectively?

- Many investigators have failed to reach goals in recruiting, enrolling and retaining racial and ethnic minority groups in research studies and clinical trials. Studies that will clarify the barriers to reaching, recruiting, enrolling and retaining racial and ethnic minorities in Alzheimer's disease research proposals are sought. The studies should also test procedures to eliminate the barriers and enhance recruitment, retention and satisfaction.
- Direct interventions aimed at improving the cognitive state of the person with Alzheimer's disease are needed. The goal is to shift the downward slope of the functional decline curve.
- What daily activities for persons with Alzheimer's disease are most supportive of independence and function at what stage of the disease? How do these activities vary be previous history of the person with Alzheimer's disease and with cultural expectations?
- Assisted living environments are increasingly popular for persons with Alzheimer's disease. Evaluation research detailing the characteristics of high quality assisted living environments producing specific outcomes is needed. If these environments are successful in producing positive outcomes for people with the disease, does this success directly translate to all cultural and ethnic groups?
- An estimated 23 % of the adult population is functionally illiterate in the U.S. and unable to read medical directions. Illiteracy rates vary by minority and ethnic groups. The impact for medical care, informal and institutional care and the risks presented by illiteracy must be understood. Programs for addressing the issues and risks for the illiterate person with Alzheimer's disease must be designed and tested.

Conclusions

Enormous strides have been made in the neurobiology of aging and in the diseases of later life, particularly Alzheimer's disease. The upcoming decades offer unparalleled promise for the dramatic expansion of neurobiological research, for unraveling the mechanisms of the disease and for the development of treatments and preventive interventions. However, the heterogeneity of the new upcoming cohorts of people with Alzheimer's disease and their families will present important challenges to investigators, clinicians and service providers.

The Epidemiology of Alzheimer's Disease: The Role of Estrogen in Reducing Risk

*V. W. Henderson**

Summary

Dementia due to Alzheimer's disease is among the most feared accompaniments of aging. There is a strong biological rationale for the use of estrogen replacement after the menopause to help reduce a woman's risk of Alzheimer's disease. Women with this disorder are less likely to use estrogens than control subjects and, among women with Alzheimer's disease, those who use estrogen perform better on cognitive tasks than those who do not. The strongest data on Alzheimer's prevention are based on case-control and cohort studies in which information on estrogen use was collected prospectively, before the onset of dementia symptoms. Studies from the Leisure World retirement community in southern California, New York City, Baltimore, and Rochester, Minnesota, imply that estrogen replacement therapy is associated with Alzheimer's risk reductions of about one-third to one-half. In several studies, a dose-response relationship has been observed, such that women who have greater estrogen exposures (higher doses or longer durations of therapy) also have lower risks of developing Alzheimer's disease. An association between Alzheimer's disease and estrogen has not been discerned in all studies, however. In the future, the role of estrogen will best be determined from results of properly designed randomized, placebo-controlled, primary prevention trials of estrogen.

Introduction

The pathogenesis of Alzheimer's disease, the most prevalent cause of dementia, is unknown. It is apparent, however, that different genetic and nongenetic factors – several of which have now been identified – can in isolation or combination culminate in the characteristic clinical and neuropathological phenotype of Alzheimer's disease. Point mutations in genes on chromosomes 14, 1, and 21 are expressed as autosomal dominant traits, with symptoms of dementia by the fifth or sixth decades of life (Pericak-Vance and Haines 1995). However, these rare

* Department of Neurology, University of Southern California School of Medicine, 1420 San Pablo Street, Suite PMB-B105, Los Angeles, California 90033, United States.
Tel 323-442-1230, Fax 323-442-1231.

R. Mayeux / Y. Christen (Eds.)
Epidemiology of Alzheimer's Disease:
From Gene to Prevention

mutations do not play an important role in the illness that first appears after about age 60 (so-called late-onset Alzheimer's disease), where it is likely that a number of "susceptibility" genes modify risk in a less deterministic manner. The best characterized of these is the chromosome 19 gene that encodes for apolipoprotein E, a lipid transport protein involved in neuronal repair (Poirier 1994). Increased Alzheimer's susceptibility is conferred by possession of the ε4 allele (Strittmatter et al. 1993), which in Alzheimer's patients is associated with deficient neuronal plasticity (Arendt et al. 1997). Gender appears to modify risk, with the ε4 allele increasing risk to a greater extent for women than men (Poirier et al. 1993; Payami et al. 1996).

As reviewed by Graves and Kukull (1994) and Breteler et al. (1992), a number of other factors modify risk. Elevated risk is thought to be associated with increasing age, low educational attainment, female gender, prior head injury, or prior episodes of depression. Although controversial, there is also evidence that risk is decreased by exposure to anti-inflammatory medications, nicotine and, among women, the use of estrogen replacement therapy after the menopause.

Estrogen and Alzheimer's Risk

Of the putative protective factors for Alzheimer's disease, estrogen replacement therapy has been the best studied. In its most explicit form, the estrogen hypothesis states that a woman's use of estrogen replacement therapy will reduce her risk of subsequent dementia due to Alzheimer's disease. A causal link between estrogen therapy and lowered Alzheimer's risk would be most firmly established if 1) the inferred link is biologically credible, 2) estrogen exposure is known to have occurred before the onset of disease and the association is strong (as indicated by a very low relative risk), 3) there is a dose-response relationship between estrogen exposure and the reduction of Alzheimer's risk, and 4) there is consistency in findings among various analytical studies of estrogen and Alzheimer's risk as well as among investigations of estrogen effects in other clinical settings relevant to the estrogen hypothesis (Hennekens and Buring 1987).

Biological Credibility of the Estrogen Hypothesis

Menopause, with the concomitant loss of ovarian estrogen production (Jaffe 1991), occurs at a mean age of about 51 years. In the absence of hormone replacement, a woman will therefore spend about 40 % of her adult life in a state of relative estrogen deprivation. The brain is an important estrogen target organ. Although the neurophysiological consequences of estrogen deprivation are poorly understood, a number of estrogen actions are potentially relevant to Alzheimer's disease (Table 1; Henderson 1997 a). Within the brain, an estrogen molecule (e.g., estradiol) will bond with a specific intranuclear receptor. After homodimerization, the paired receptor-ligand complex binds to a particular DNA

Table 1. Biological Actions of Estrogen that Are Potentially Relevant to Alzheimer's Disease[a]

- Effects on the growth, differentiation, and survival of nerve cells
- Effects on synapse formation
- Effects on glial cells
- Effects on actylcholine and other neurotransmitter systems
- Decreased formation of the β-amyloid protein
- Increased expression of apolipoprotein E in the brain
- Antioxidant actions
- Anti-inflammatory actions
- Blunted cortisol response to behavioral stress
- Increased cerebral blood flow
- Increased transport of glucose into the brain

[a] Adapted from Henderson (1997 a).

sequence to regulate the synthesis of a specific protein product. Other estrogen actions, some of which involve pharmacologically characterized membrane receptors, do not require interactions with the genome (Kawata 1995; Wong et al. 1996).

Through genomic and nongenomic mechanisms, estrogen influences the activity of various neurotransmitter systems. A coherent body of experimental and clinical evidence supports the importance of acetylcholine in attention and memory (Bartus et al. 1981), and the current mainstay of the pharmacological treatment of Alzheimer's disease seeks to increase levels of this particular neurotransmitter. In the Alzheimer brain, characteristic pathological aggregates (neurofibrillary tangles) accumulate within cholinergic neurons of the basal forebrain region (Coyle et al. 1983). These neurons possess receptors for estrogen (Toran-Allerand et al. 1992), and in the laboratory estrogen treatment elevates cholinergic markers in the basal forebrain and in projection target areas (Luine 1985; Gibbs and Pfaff 1992). Cholinergic neurons within the basal forebrain also have receptors for neurotrophins, and estrogen may modulate neurotrophin effects (Toran-Allerand et al. 1992; Miranda et al. 1993; Salehi et al. 1996). Indirect evidence that estrogen interacts with cholinergic neurons comes from a clinical trial of Alzheimer's patients treated with an inhibitor of the enzyme acetylcholinesterase. In this trial, the cognitive skills of women receiving estrogen and randomized to the anticholinesterase group were significantly better than those of women given placebo; however, women not receiving estrogen and randomized to active drug performed more like the placebo group (Schneider et al. 1996).

Estrogen interacts with other neurotransmitters disrupted by Alzheimer's pathology. Both locus ceruleus and raphe neurons are prominently affected by neurofibrillary tangle formation. Locus ceruleus neurons, which provide widespread noradrenergic input to different brain areas, have estrogen receptors (Sar and Stumpf 1981). Widely projecting serotonergic neurons in the brain stem raphe are also influenced by estrogen (Greengrass and Tonge 1974; Biegon et al. 1983; Sumner and Fink 1995).

Estrogen is both neurotrophic and neuroprotective. Estrogen promotes the outgrowth of neurites in primary of brain (Toran-Allerand 1991; Brinton et al. 1997), axonal sprouting after experimental brain lesions (Morse et al. 1986), and the formation of synapses (Chung et al. [1988]; Woolley and McEwen 1992). Astroglia, like neurons, can undergo morphological alterations in response to estrogen exposure (Garcia-Segura et al. 1997).

Estrogens might reduce formation of the β-amyloid protein (Xu et al. 1998). In the Alzheimer's brain, this abnormal protein fragment is deposited in neuritic plaques, located in the neuropil of the gray matter. There is also a link between estrogens and apolipoprotein E. Apolipoprotein E levels are reduced in the cerebrospinal fluid (Blennow et al. 1994) and brain (Bertrand et al. 1995) of Alzheimer's patients. Estrogen, however, acts to increase the expression of central nervous system apolipoprotein E (Stone et al. 1997), which might facilitate neuronal repair. In animal models, estrogen-dependent neuronal sprouting after experimental lesions (Morse et al. 1986) requires the presence of apolipoprotein E (Stone et al. 1998).

The effects of estrogen on the immune system might favorably impact Alzheimer's disease. Anti-inflammatory medications are postulated to reduce Alzheimer's risk (Rich et al. 1995) and to improve dementia symptoms (Rogers et al. 1993). Estrogen moderates some aspects of the inflammatory process (Pacifici et al. 1991; Josefsson et al. 1992).

Estrogen may protect neurons from programmed cell death (apoptosis) and from death due to oxidative stress, excitatory neurotoxicity, ischemia, and other insults (Goodman et al. 1996; Singer et al. 1996; Behl et al. 1997; Regan and Guo 1997; Simpkins et al. 1997). There is prominent indication of oxidative damage in Alzheimer's disease brain (Smith et al. 1997), and the antioxidant α-tocopherol (vitamin E) is reported to retard the clinical course of Alzheimer's disease (Sano et al. 1997). Neuronal damage attributed to the β-amyloid protein may be mediated or potentiated by free radicals (Sagara et al. 1996; McDonald et al. 1997). Antioxidant properties of estrogens (Mooradian 1993; Sack et al. 1994) might therefore serve a protective role in Alzheimer's disease.

Corticosteroid secretion is increased by behavioral stress and can deleteriously affect hippocampal neurons (McEwen and Sapolsky 1995). Basal cortisol levels are reported to be elevated in Alzheimer's disease (Davis et al. 1986), and estrogen replacement therapy may mitigate the stress response in older women (Lindheim et al. 1992).

Estrogen increases regional blood flow within the brain (Belfort et al. 1995; Ohkura et al. 1995). It also increases the uptake of glucose into the brain by increasing the expression of a glucose transporter protein within the blood-brain barrier (Shi and Simpkins 1997).

Timing of Exposure and Strength of Exposure

If estrogen therapy protects against Alzheimer's disease, then one would expect that estrogen would be used less often by women with Alzheimer's disease than by other women. This prediction has been supported in recent studies of late-onset Alzheimer's cases. In 1994, Birge noted that none of the 158 women in his Alzheimer's clinic were current estrogen users. That same year, as part of a longitudinal study of aging and dementia, Henderson et al. (1994) in Los Angeles compared 143 women with Alzheimer's disease and 92 healthy women without dementia (mean age 76 years in both groups). Eighteen percent of controls but only seven percent of Alzheimer's cases used estrogen. The two groups were similar in terms of other medication use and surgical procedures likely to influence the prescription of estrogen. However, differences in estrogen usage were significant (the estimate of relative risk, or odds ratio [OR] was 0.33, and the 95 % confidence interval [CI] was 0.15 to 0.74.) Similar results were described in cross-sectional analyses by Mortel and Meyer (1995) in Houston, who compared 93 clinic cases to a convenience sample of 148 controls (OR = 0.55, 95 % CI = 0.26 to 1.26). Although analyses based on current estrogen use imply substantial risk reductions, results must be interpreted cautiously. Most important among several methodological limitations is the fact that it was not ascertained to what extent women were exposed to estrogen during the time of interest, i. e., in the years before the onset of dementia symptoms. If demented women are more likely to be prescribed estrogen, the resulting bias would underestimate the magnitude of any protective effect. Conversely, if estrogen prescriptions were more likely to be discontinued among Alzheimer's cases, then a protective effect might be inferred in the absence of any true effect or the magnitude of a true protective effect could be overestimated.

Prior (ever versus never) estrogen exposure had been considered in earlier case-control studies from the United States (Heyman et al. 1984; Graves et al. 1990), Italy (Amaducci et al. 1986) and Australia (Broe et al. 1990). These failed to discern a significant relation between estrogen exposure and Alzheimer's risk (ORs ranged from 0.48 to 2.48), although the low proportion of women who actually used estrogen (ranging from 8 % to 16 % exposure within the control groups) and relatively small sample sizes limited statistical power. Recent case-control studies are more supportive of the estrogen hypothesis. Lerner et al. (1997) in Cleveland found that Alzheimer's cases were less likely than controls to have used estrogen in the past (OR = 0.58, 95 % CI = 0.25 to 0.91), as did Van Duijn et al. (1996) in a European population-based study of early-onset disease (OR = 0.40, 95 % CI = 0.19 to 0.91; but see below). In a large population-based Italian study, Baldereschi et al. (1998) found reduced estrogen usage among 92 Alzheimer's cases (mean age at onset of 75 years) in comparison to 1476 women without dementia (OR = 0.28, 95 % CI = 0.08 to 0.98).

In some case-control studies (Birge 1994; Henderson et al. 1994; Mortel and Meyer 1995; Lerner et al. 1997; Baldereschi et al. 1998), recall bias might have occurred when information on estrogen exposure was obtained differently for an

Alzheimer's case (e.g. from a surrogate informant) than for a control (e.g., from the woman herself). Other recent analyses, however, have relied on estrogen exposure data collected prospectively, before the onset of dementia symptoms (Paganini-Hill and Henderson 1994, 1996; Brenner et al. 1994; Tang et al. 1996; Kawas et al. 1997; Waring et al. 1997). The largest such study (Paganini-Hill and Henderson 1994, 1996) is from the Leisure World retirement community, a predominantly White upper middle class cohort in southern California that was established by postal survey in the early 1980s. Information on estrogen therapy in this defined cohort was collected from each woman at the time of enrollment. Death certificate records were subsequently obtained for deceased participants. For female cohort members who died before 1996, Paganini-Hill and Henderson (1996) identified 248 Alzheimer's disease cases (mean age at death 88 years) and 1198 matched controls. In this nested case-control study, estrogen users had a one-third lower risk of Alzheimer's disease (OR = 0.65, 95 % CI = 0.49 to 0.88). Different routes of estrogen administration (oral, oral plus injection or cream, injection or cream) were each associated with significant risk reductions. In Leisure World, cases were not examined in person, and death records almost certainly missed some Alzheimer's cases; however, misclassification was most likely nondifferential with respect to estrogen exposure, and the resulting risk estimates may therefore have underestimated the association between estrogen therapy and Alzheimer's risk reduction.

Results similar to those described in Leisure World are reported from New York, Baltimore, and Rochester, Minnesota, where case ascertainment included in-person medical assessments. In an ethnically diverse community-based cohort from the northern Manhattan section of New York City, Tang et al. (1996), identified 167 incident cases of Alzheimer's disease (mean age 79 years). There was a 50 % risk reduction of Alzheimer's disease among women who had used oral estrogens after the menopause (OR = 0.5, 95 % CI = 0.25 to 0.9). Moreover, these investigators observed a significantly older age at onset among women who had used estrogen than among other Alzheimer's cases. Significant risk reductions were found both for women who possessed the ε4 allele of apolipoprotein E as well as for women without this allele. In contrast, apolipoprotein E polymorphisms appeared to modify the effect of estrogen exposure among early-onset cases of familial Alzheimer's disease reported by van Duijn et al. (1996), where a protective effect of estrogen was apparent only among women with the ε4 allele.

In the Baltimore Longitudinal Study of Aging, Kawas and her colleagues (1997) identified 34 incident cases of Alzheimer's disease among 472 older women. The risk of this illness was reduced by over a half when women who had used oral or transdermal estrogen were compared to never-users (OR = 0.46, 95 % CI = 0.209 to 0.997). In a preliminary analysis from Rochester, Minnesota, Waring et al. (1997) analyzed medical records of 222 women who developed Alzheimer's disease during a five-year interval. Compared to matched controls without dementia, cases were significantly less likely to have used estrogen for at least six months (OR = 0.4, 95 % CI = 0.2 to 0.8).

In contrast to these positive studies, a case-control analysis of subjects derived from a health maintenance organization cohort in the Puget Sound region of Washington showed no relation between estrogen use and Alzheimer's risk (Brenner et al. 1994). As had investigators from Leisure World, New York, Baltimore, and Rochester, Brenner et al. (1994) documented estrogen use prospectively. They used computerized pharmacy records to compare estrogen exposure between 107 incident cases of Alzheimer's disease (mean age 79 years) and 120 frequency-matched controls. Receiving a prescription for estrogen did not affect the risk of subsequent Alzheimer's disease (OR = 1.1, 95 % CI = 0.6 to 1.8); a post hoc analyses that considered only prescriptions for oral estrogen found a non-significant risk reduction (OR = 0.7, 95 % CI = 0.4 to 1.5).

Dose-Response Relationship

Several epidemiological studies have provided information on the magnitude of estrogen exposure and Alzheimer's risk. In Leisure World, risk estimates for Alzheimer's disease decreased significantly with larger doses of the longest used oral

Table 2. Effect of Estrogen Dosage in the Leisure World Cohort: Risk Estimates for Alzheimer's Disease as a Function of Dosage for the Longest Used Oral Estrogen Preparation[a]

Dosage (mg)	Number of cases	Number of controls	Odds ratio	95 % Confidence interval	Probability (trend test)
none	150	615	1.00	–	< 0.01
≤ 0.625	27	141	0.78	0.48–1.27	
≥ 1.25	21	156	0.54	0.32–0.92	

[a] Data are from Paganini-Hill and Henderson (1996).

Table 3. Risk Estimates for Alzheimer's Disease as a Function of the Duration of Postmenopausal Estrogen Therapy in Three Epidemiological Studies

Study/authors	Estrogen preparations(s)	Duration of use (years)	Odds ratio	95 % Confidence interval	Probability
Leisure World/ Paganini-Hill and Henderson (1996)	All	Never	1.00	–	< 0.001
		≤ 3	0.83	0.56–1.22	
		4–14	0.50	0.31–0.81	
		≥ 15	0.44	0.26–0.75	
New York/ Tang et al. (1996)	Oral	Never	1.00	–	0.003
		≤ 1	0.47	0.20–1.10	
		> 1	0.13	0.02–0.92	
Baltimore/ Kawas et al. (1997)	Oral/patch	Never	1.00	–	NS[a]
		≤ 5	0.43	0.13–1.51	
		6–10	0.34	0.04–2.52	
		≥ 11	0.50	0.17–1.47	

[a] NS, not significant.

estrogen preparation (Paganini-Hill and Henderson 1996; Table 2). Significant associations between the duration of estrogen use and the degree of risk reduction were noted both in Leisure World (Paganini-Hill and Henderson 1996) and New York (Tang et al. 1996), but no significant trend was discerned in the Baltimore study (Kawas et al. 1997; (Table 3). In Rochester, Minnesota, risk decreased with increasing duration of estrogen use and with increasing total cumulative dose (Waring et al. 1997), and in Puget Sound women who filled the largest number of estrogen prescriptions experienced the lowest Alzheimer's risk (Brenner et al. 1994).

Consistency of Findings: Surrogate Markers of Estrogen Exposure and Alzheimer's Risk

After the menopause, circulating estrogens are derived primarily from the peripheral conversion of androgen precursors produced by the ovarian stroma and the adrenal cortex. Much of the extraglandular conversion occurs in adipose tissue, and body weight in older women therefore correlates with estrogen levels (Meldrum et al. 1981). In Leisure World, body weight at the time of cohort enrollment was significantly associated with a subsequent Alzheimer's diagnosis (Paganini-Hill and Henderson 1996), but there was no relation between retrospective estimates of body weight at age 50 years and prevalent cases of Alzheimer's disease in the Italian Longitudinal Study on Aging (Baldereschi et al. 1998).

Reproductive factors that may increase endogenous estrogen exposure include earlier age at menarche, parity (or number of pregnancies), and later age at menopause. Analyses of these variables provide only weak support for the estrogen hypothesis. In both Leisure World (Paganini-Hell and Henderson 1996) and the Italian study (Baldereschi et al. 1998), an earlier age at menarche was associated with a lower risk of Alzheimer's disease, but neither study found parity to be related to Alzheimer's risk. In Rochester, the median age at menarche was similar for both cases and controls (Waring et al. 1997). Moreover, there is no support for the contention that a later menopause protects against late-onset Alzheimer's disease (Baldereschi et al. 1998; Paganini-Hill and Henderson 1996; Tang et al. 1996; Waring et al. 1997), although in one study early menopause was associated with increased risk of early-onset illness in women with a positive family history (van Duijn et al. 1996).

Consistency of Findings: Clinical Studies in Women Without Dementia

The view that estrogen modulates neural activity related to cognition is supported by a brain imaging study undertaken while women performed a specific neuropsychological task (Berman et al. 1997). The pattern of activation was found to differ, depending on a woman's hormonal status (estrogen deficient versus estrogen replenished). An estrogen effect on cognition is also implied by cognitive fluctuations during a woman's menstrual cycle (Hampson 1990; Phillips and Sherwin 1992 a; Krug et al. 1994; Bibawi et al. 1995), by neuropsychological dysfunction after the suppression of endogenous estrogen production and improvement after the administration of exogenous estrogen (Varney et al. 1993; Sherwin and Tulandi 1996); and by enhanced test scores in women receiving estrogen replacement after the menopause (Kampen and Sherwin 1994; Robinson et al. 1994; Phillips and Sherwin 1992 b).

In a population-based cohort in Austria, cross-sectional analyses showed that estrogen users outperformed nonusers on measures of psychomotor speed and complex problem solving (Schmidt et al. 1996). Findings from two well-characterized American cohorts suggest that estrogen replacement therapy protects against longitudinal decline in several cognitive domains (Resnick et al. 1997; Jacobs et al. 1998), although two other American studies found no compelling evidence that estrogen preserved cognitive function among older women (Barrett-Connor and Kritz-Silverstein 1993; Szklo et al. 1996).

Consistency of Findings: Clinical Studies in Women with Dementia

Observational analyses by Henderson et al. (1996) imply that women with Alzheimer's disease who are prescribed estrogen perform better on a variety of cognitive tasks than Alzheimer's patients not receiving hormone replacement. In their study, differences favoring estrogen-users were greatest on a naming (semantic memory) task, the same cognitive task that was found to be more impaired among women than men with Alzheimer's disease (Henderson and Buckwalter 1994; Ripich et al. 1995).

Several clinical trials have examined the effects of oral or transdermal estrogen on cognitive symptoms of women with Alzheimer's disease; most results suggest that estrogen ameliorates Alzheimer's symptoms (Henderson 1997 b). Four of these studies have been conducted as randomized, placebo-controlled trials (Honjo et al. 1993; Fillit 1994; Asthana et al. 1996; Birge 1997), although only the study of Honjo et al. (1993) has been fully presented. Positive results in most of these trials provides preliminary evidence that estrogen improves cognitive function in Alzheimer's disease, and results thus indirectly support the parallel contention that estrogen could also help prevent Alzheimer's disease. Results of larger randomized, placebo-controlled trials are anticipated within a year's time. Additional indirect evidence for an estrogen role comes from a study by Buckwalter et al. (1997) that examined body weight in relation to cognitive symptoms in women with Alzheimer's disease. In analyses that adjusted for age, education, symptom duration, and height, greater body weight in women with Alzheimer's disease was linked to significantly better performance on tests of cognitive ability.

Conclusions

A strong biological rationale supports the contention that estrogen could impact brain functions involved in cognition and physiological processes implicated in the pathogenesis or progression of Alzheimer's disease. The hypothesis that estrogen protects against Alzheimer's disease finds partial support from observational and clinical studies on indirect markers of estrogen exposure, cognition in healthy women, and cognition in women with Alzheimer's disease.

Over a dozen case-control and cohort studies have now examined the relation between estrogen usage and Alzheimer's risk. In most reports, the temporal relation between exposure and outcome is unambiguous; in these it is clear that estrogen therapy was indeed prescribed prior to the onset of dementia symptoms. With important exceptions (Brenner et al. 1994), epidemiological investigations since 1990 are also consistent in indicating a protective effect of estrogen. If confirmed, the magnitude of risk reduction in these studies (approximately one third to one half) would be of enormous public health importance. However, the magnitude is not so large that alternative interpretations should not still be considered. Because women who receive estrogen replacement differ in important ways from women who do not use estrogen (Hemminki et al. 1993; Derby et al. 1995), it is prudent to consider the possibility that residual confounding or unrecognized biases may account for observed associations.

Consistent findings in future cohort studies – especially those that are population-based – would strengthen the argument for a causal link between estrogen therapy and reduced Alzheimer's risk. The strongest support, however, will come from adequately powered randomized, placebo-controlled intervention trials. In the United States, it is anticipated that over 7500 older women will be randomized in an ancillary study of dementia, undertaken in conjunction with the Women's Health Initiative and sponsored by the National Institutes of Health. Results of this primary prevention study, which involves the randomized use of oral estrogens, will not be available until after the millennium. Other randomized trials are also anticipated during the next several years.

References

Amaducci LA, Fratiglioni L, Rocca WA, Fieschi C, Livrea P, Pedone D, Bracco L, Lippi A, Grandolfo C, Bino G, Prencipe M, Bonatti ML, Girotti F, Carella F, Tavolato B, Ferla S, Lenzi GL, Carolei A, Gambi A, Grigoletto F, Schoenberg BS (1986) Risk factors for clinically diagnosed Alzheimer's disease: a case-control study of an Italian population. Neurology 36:922–931

Arendt T, Schindler C, Brückner MK, Eschrich K, Bigl V, Zedlick D, Marcova L (1997) Plastic neuronal remodeling is impaired in patients with Alzheimer's disease carrying apolipoprotein ε4 allele. J Neurosci 17:516–529

Asthana S, Craft S, Baker LD, Raskind MA, Avery E, Lofgreen C, Wilkinson CW, Falzgraf S, Veith RC, Plymate SR (1996) Transdermal estrogen improves memory in women with Alzheimer's disease [abstract]. Soc Neurosci Abstr 22:200

Baldereschi M, Di Carlo A, Lepore V, Bracco L, Maggi S, Grigoletto F, Scarlato G, Amaducci L (1998) Estrogen-replacement therapy and Alzheimer's disease in the Italian Longitudinal Study on Aging. Neurology 50: 996–1002

Barrett-Connor E, Kritz-Silverstein D (1993) Estrogen replacement therapy and cognitive function in older women. JAMA 269:2637–2641

Bartus RT, Dean RL, Beer B, Lippa AD (1981) The cholinergic hypothesis of geriatric memory dysfunction. Science 217:208–217

Behl C, Skutella T, Lezoualch F, Post A, Widmann M, Newton CJ, Holsboer F (1997) Neuroprotection against oxidative stress by estrogens: structure-activity relationship. Mol Pharmacol 51:535–541

Belfort MA, Saade GR, Snabes M, Dunn R, Moise KJ, Jr, Cruz A, Young R (1995) Hormonal status affects the reactivity of the cerebral vasculature. Am J Obstet Gynecol 172:1273–1278

Berman KF, Schmidt PJ, Rubinow DR, Danaceau MA, Van Horn JD, Esposito G, Ostrem JL, Weinberger DR (1997) Modulation of cognition-specific cortical activity by gonadal steroids: a positron-emission tomography study in women. Proc Natl Acad Sci USA 94:8836–8841

Bertrand P, Poirier J, Oda T, Finch CE, Pasinetti GM (1995) Association of apolipoprotein E genotype with brain levels of apolipoprotein E and apolipoprotein J (clusterin) in Alzheimer disease. Mol Brain Res 33:174–178

Bibawi D, Cherry B, Hellige JB (1995) Fluctuations of perceptual asymmetry across time in women and men: effects related to the menstrual cycle. Neuropsychologia 33: 131–138

Biegon A, Reches A, Snyder L, McEwen BS (1983) Serotonergic and noradrenergic receptors in the rat brain: modulation by chronic exposure to ovarian hormones. Life Sci 32:2015–2021

Birge SJ (1994) The role of estrogen deficiency in the aging central nervous system. In: Lobo RA (ed) Treatment of the postmenopausal woman: basic and clinical aspects. Raven Press, New York, pp 153–157

Birge SJ (1997) The role of estrogen in the treatment of Alzheimer's disease. Neurology 48 [suppl. 7]:S36–S41

Blennow K, Hesse C, Fredman P (1994) Cerebrospinal fluid apolipoprotein E is reduced in Alzheimer's disease. NeuroReport 5:2534–2536

Brenner DE, Kukull WA, Stergachis A, van Belle G, Bowen JD, McCormick WC, Teri L, Larson EB (1994) Postmenopausal estrogen replacement therapy and the risk of Alzheimer's disease: a population-based case-control study. Am J Epidemiol 140: 262–267

Breteler MMB, Claus JJ, van Duijn CM, Launer LJ, Hofman A (1992) Epidemiology of Alzheimer's disease. Epidemiol Rev 14:59–82

Brinton RD, Tran J, Proffitt P, Montoya M (1997) 17 β-estradiol enhances the outgrowth and survival of neocortical neurons in culture. Neurochem Res 22:1339–1351

Broe GA, Henderson AS, Creasey H, McCusker E, Korten AE, Jorm AF, Longley W, Anthony JC (1990) A case-control study of Alzheimer's disease in Australia. Neurology 40:1698–1707

Buckwalter JG, Schneider LS, Wilshire TW, Dunn ME, Henderson VW (1997) Body weight, estrogen and cognitive functioning in Alzheimer's disease: an analysis of the tacrine study group. Arch Gerontol Geriatr 24:261–267

Chung SK, Pfaff DW, Cohen RS (1988) Estrogen-induced alterations in synaptic morphology in the midbrain central gray. Exp Brain Res 69:522–530

Coyle JT, Price DL, DeLong MR (1983) Alzheimer's disease: a disorder of cortical cholinergic innervation. Science 219:1184–1190

Davis KL, Davis BM, Greenwald BS, Mohs RC, Mathé AA, Johns CA, Horvath TB (1986) Cortisol and Alzheimer's disease. Am J Psych 143:300–305

Derby CA, Hume AL, McPhillips JB, Barbour MM, Carleton RA (1995) Prior and current health characteristics of postmenopausal estrogen replacement therapy users compared with nonusers. Am J Obstet Gynecol 173:544–550

Fillit H (1994) Estrogens in the pathogenesis and treatment of Alzheimer's disease in postmenopausal women. Ann N Y Acad Sci 743:233–238

Garcia-Segura LM, Chowen JA, Dueñas M, Parducz A, Naftolin F (1997) Gonadal steroids and astroglial plasticity. Cell Mol Neurobiol 16: 225–237

Gibbs RB, Pfaff DW (1992) Effects of estrogen and fimbria/fornix transection on $p75^{NGFR}$ and ChAT expression in the medial septum and diagonal band of Broca. Exp. Neurol 116:23–39

Goodman Y, Bruce AJ, Cheng B, Mattson MP (1996) Estrogens attenuate and corticosterone exacerbates excitotoxicity, oxidative injury, and amyloid β-peptide toxicity in hippocampal neurons. J Neurochem 66: 1836–1844

Graves AB, Kukull WA (1994) The epidemiology of dementia. In: Morris JC (ed) Handbook of dementing illnesses. Marcel Dekker, New York, pp 23–69

Graves AB, White E, Koepsell TD, Reifler BV, van Belle G, Larson EB, Raskind M (1990) A case-control study of Alzheimer's disease. Ann Neurol 28:766–774

Greengrass PM, Tonge SR (1974) The accumulation of noradrenaline and 5-hydroxytryptamine in three regions of mouse brain after tetrabenazine and iproniazid: effects of ethinyloestradiol and progesterone. Psychopharmacologia 39:187–191

Hampson E (1990) Variations in sex-related cognitive abilities across the menstrual cycle. Brain Cognit 14:26–43

Hemminki E, Malin M, Topo P (1993) Selection to postmenopausal therapy by women's characteristics. J Clin Epidemiol 46:211–219

Henderson VW (1997 a) Estrogen, cognition, and a woman's risk of Alzheimer's disease. Am J Med 103[suppl. 3 A]:11–18

Henderson VW (1997 b) Estrogen replacement therapy for the prevention and treatment of Alzheimer's disease. CNS Drugs 8:343–351

Henderson VW, Buckwalter JG (1994) Cognitive deficits of men and women with Alzheimer's disease. Neurology 44:90–96

Henderson VW, Paganini-Hill A, Emanuel CK, Dunn ME, Buckwalter JG (1994) Estrogen replacement therapy in older women: comparisons between Alzheimer's disease cases and nondemented control subjects. Arch Neurol 51:896–900

Henderson VW, Watt L, Buckwalter JG (1996) Cognitive skills associated with estrogen replacement in women with Alzheimer's disease. Psychoneuroendocrinology 21:421–430

Hennekens CH, Buring JE (1987) Epidemiology in medicine. Little Brown and Company, Boston

Heyman A, Wilkinson WE, Stafford JA, Helms JJ, Sigmon AH, Weinberg T (1984) Alzheimer's disease: a study of epidemiological aspects. Ann Neurol 15:335–341

Honjo H, Ogino Y, Tanaka K, Urabe M, Kashiwagi T, Ishihara S, Okada H, Araki K, Fushiki S, Nakajima K, Hayashi K, Hayashi M, Sakaki T (1993) An effect of conjugated estrogen to cognitive impairment in women with senile dementia – Alzheimer's type: a placebo-controlled double blind study. J Jpn Menopause Soc 1:167–171

Jacobs DM, Tang MX, Stern Y, Sano M, Marder K, Bell KL, Schofield P, Dooneief G, Gurland B, Mayeux R (1998) Cognitive function in nondemented older women who took estrogen after menopause. Neurology 50:368–373

Jaffe RB (1991) The menopause and perimenopausal period. In: Yen SSC, Jaffe RB (eds) Reproductive endocrinology, 3rd Ed. WB Saunders, Philadelphia, pp 389–408

Josefsson E, Tarkowski A, Carlsten H (1992) Anti-inflammatory properties of estrogen. Cell Immunol 142:67–78

Kampen DL, Sherwin BB (1994) Estrogen use and verbal memory in healthy postmenopausal women. Obstet Gynecol 83:979–983

Kawas C, Resnick S, Morrison A, Brookmeyer R, Corrada M, Zonderman A, Bacal C, Donnell Lingle D, Metter E (1997) A prospective study of estrogen replacement therapy and the risk of developing Alzheimer's disease: the Baltimore Longitudinal Study of Aging. Neurology 48:1517–1521

Kawata M (1995) Roles of steroid hormones and their receptors in structural organization in the nervous system. Neurosci Res 24:1–46

Krug R, Stamm U, Pietrowsky R, Fehm HL, Born J (1994) Effects of menstrual cycle on creativity. Psychoneuroendocrinology 19:21–31

Lerner A, Koss E, Debanne S, Rowland D, Smyth K, Friedland R (1997) Smoking and oestrogen-replacement therapy as protective factors for Alzheimer's disease [letter]. Lancet 349:403–404

Lindheim SR, Legro RS, Bernstein L, Stanczyk FZ, Vijod MA, Presser SC, Lobo RA (1992) Behavioral stress responses in premenopausal and postmenopausal women and the effects of estrogen. Am J Obstet Gynecol 167:1831–1836

Luine V (1985) Estradiol increases choline acetyltransferase activity in specific basal forebrain nuclei and projection areas of female rats. Exp Neurol 89:484–490

McDonald DR, Brunden KR, Landreth GE (1997) Amyloid fibrils activate tyrosine kinase-dependent signaling and superoxide production in microglia. J Neurosci 17: 2284–2294

McEwen BS, Sapolsky RM (1995) Stress and cognitive function. Curr Opin Neurobiol 5:205–216

Meldrum DR, Davidson BJ, Tataryn IV, Judd HL (1981) Changes in circulating steroids with aging in postmenopausal women. Obstet Gynecol 57:624–628

Miranda RC, Sohrabji F, Toran-Allerand CD (1993) Presumptive estrogen target neurons express mRNAs for both the neurotrophins and neurotrophin receptors: a basis for potential developmental interactions of estrogen with neurotrophins. Mol Cell Neurosci 4:510–525

Mooradian AD (1993) Antioxidant properties of steroids. J Steroid Biochem Mol Biol 45:509–511

Morse JD, Scheff SW, DeKosky ST (1986) Gonadal steroids influence axon sprouting in the hippocampal dentate gyrus: a sexually dimorphic response. Exp Neurol 94:649–658

Mortel KF, Meyer JS (1995) Lack of postmenopausal estrogen replacement therapy and the risk of dementia. J Neuropsychiatr Clin Neurosci 7:334–337

Ohkura T, Teshima Y, Isse K, Matsuda H, Inoue T, Sakai Y, Iwasaki N, Yoshimasa Y (1995) Estrogen increases cerebral and cerebellar blood flows in postmenopausal women. Menopause 2:13–18

Pacifici R, Brown C, Puscheck E, Friedrich E, Slatopolsky E, Maggio D, McCracken R, Avioli LV (1991) Effect of surgical menopause and estrogen replacement on cytokine release from human blood mononuclear cells. Proc Natl Acad Sci USA 88:5134–5138

Paganini-Hill A, Henderson VW (1994) Estrogen deficiency and risk of Alzheimer's disease in women. Am J Epidemiol 140:256–261

Paganini-Hill A, Henderson VW (1996) Estrogen replacement therapy and risk of Alzheimer's disease. Arch Intern Med 156:2213–2217

Payami H, Zareparsi S, Montee KR, Sexton GJ, Kaye JA, Bird TD, Yu CE, Wijsman EM, Heston LL, Litrt M, Schellenberg GD (1996) Gender difference in apolipoprotein E-associated risk for familial Alzheimer disease: a possible clue to the higher incidence of Alzheimer disease in women. Am J Hum Genet 58:803–811

Pericak-Vance MA, Haines JL (1995) Genetic susceptibility to Alzheimer disease. Trends Genet 11:504–508

Phillips SM, Sherwin BB (1992 a) Variations in memory function and sex steroid hormones across the menstrual cycle. Psychoneuroendocrinology 17:497–506

Phillips SM, Sherwin BB (1992 b) Effects of estrogen on memory function in surgically menopausal women. Psychoneuroendocrinology 17:485–495

Poirier J (1994) Apolipoprotein E in animal models of CNS injury and in Alzheimer's disease. Trends Neurosci 17:525–530

Poirier J, Davignon J, Bouthillier D, Kogan S, Bertrand P, Gauthier S (1993) Apolipoprotein E polymorphism and Alzheimer's disease. Lancet 342:697–699

Regan RF, Guo Y (1997) Estrogens attenuate neuronal injury due to hemoglobin, chemical hypoxia, and excitatory amino acids in murine cortical cultures. Brain Res 764:133–140

Resnick SM, Metter EJ, Zonderman AB (1997) Estrogen replacement therapy and longitudinal decline in visual memory. A possible protective effect? Neurology 49:1491–1497

Rich JB, Rasmusson DX, Folstein MF, Carson KA, Kawas C, Brandt J (1995) Nonsteroidal anti-inflammatory drugs in Alzheimer's disease. Neurology 45:51–55

Ripich DN, Petrill SA, Whitehouse PJ, Ziol EW (1995) Gender differences in language of AD patients: a longitudinal study. Neurology 45:299–302

Robinson D, Friedman L, Marcus R, Tinklenberg J, Yesavage J (1994) Estrogen replacement therapy and memory in older women. J Am Geriatr Soc 42:919–922

Rogers J, Kirby LC, Hempelman SR, Berry DL, McGeer PL, Kazniak AW, Zalinski J, Cofield M, Mansukhani L, Willson P, Kogan F (1993) Clinical trial of indomethacin in Alzheimer's disease. Neurology 43:1609–1611

Sack MN, Rader DJ, Cannon ROI (1994) Oestrogen and inhibition of oxidation of low-density lipoproteins in postmenopausal women. Lancet 343:269–270

Sagara Y, Dargusch R, Klier FG, Schubert D, Behl C (1996) Increased antioxidant enzyme activity in amyloid β protein-resistant cells. J Neurosci 16:497–505

Salehi A, Verhaagen J, Dijkhuizen PA, Swaab DF (1996) Co-localization of high-affinity neurotrophin receptors in nucleus basalis of Meynert neurons and their differential reduction in Alzheimer's disease. Neuroscience 75:373–387

Sano M, Ernesto C, Thomas RG, Klauber MR, Schafer K, Grundman M, Woodbury P, Growdon J, Cotman CW, Pfeiffer E, Schneider LS, Thal LJ (1997) A controlled trial of selegiline, alpha-tocopherol, or both as treatment for Alzheimer's disease. N Engl J Med 336:1216–1222

Sar M, Stumpf WE (1981) Central noradrenergic neurons concentrate ^{3}H-oestradiol. Nature 289:500–502

Schmidt R, Fazekas F, Reinhart B, Kapeller P, Fazekas G, Offenbacher H, Eber B, Schumacher M, Freidl W (1996) Estrogen replacement therapy in older women: a neuropsychological and brain MRI study. J Am Geriatr Soc 44:1307–1313

Schneider LS, Farlow MR, Henderson VW, Pogoda JM (1996) Effects of estrogen replacement therapy on response to tacrine in patients with Alzheimer's disease. Neurology 46:1580–1584

Sherwin BB, Tulandi T (1996) "Add-back" estrogen reverses cognitive deficits induced by a gonadotropin-releasing hormone agonist in women with leiomyomata uteri. J Clin Endocrinol Metab 81:2545–2549

Shi J, Simpkins JW (1997) 17β-estradiol modulation of glucose transporter 1 expression in blood-brain barrier. Am J Physiol 272:E1016–E1022

Simpkins JW, Rajakumar G, Zhang Y-Q, Smipkins CE, Greenwald D, Yu CJ Bodor N, Day AL (1997) Estrogens may reduce mortality and ischemic damage caused by middle cerebral artery occlusion in the female rat. J Neurosurg 87:724–730

Singer CA, Rogers KL, Strickland TM, Dorsa DM (1996) Estrogen protects primary cortical neurons from glutamate toxicity. Neurosci Lett 212:13–16

Smith MA, Harris PLR, Sayre LM, Beckman JS, Perry G (1997) Widespread peroxynitrite-mediated damage in Alzheimer's disease. J Neurosci 17:2653–2657

Stone DJ, Rozovsky I, Morgan TE, Anderson CP, Hajian H, Finch CE (1997) Astrocytes and microglia respond to estrogen with increased apoE mRNA *in vivo* and *in vitro*. Exp Neurol 143:313–318

Stone DJ, Rozovsky I, Morgan TE, Anderson CP, Finch CE (1998) Increased synaptic spouting in response to estrogen via an apolipoprotein E dependent mechanism: implications for Alzheimer's disease. J Neurosci 18:3180–3185

Strittmatter WJ, Saunders AM, Schmechel D, Pericak-Vance M, Enghild J, Salvesen GS, Roses AD (1993) Apolipoprotein E: high-avidity binding to β-amyloid and increased frequency of type 4 allele in late-onset familial Alzheimer disease. Proc Natl Acad Sci USA 90:1977–1981

Sumner BEH, Fink G (1995) Estrogen increases the density of 5-hydroxytryptamine$_{2A}$ receptors in cerebral cortex and nucleus accumbens in the female rat. J Steroid Biochem Mol Biol 54:15–20

Szklo M, Cerhan J, Diez-Roux AV, Chambless L, Cooper L, Folsom AR, Fried LP, Knopman D, Nieto FJ (1996) Estrogen replacement therapy and cognitive functioning in the Atherosclerosis Risk in Communities (ARIC) study. Am J Epidemiol 144:1048–1057

Tang M-X, Jacobs D, Stern Y, Marder K, Schofield P, Gurland B, Andrews H, Mayeux R (1996) Effect of oestrogen during menopause on risk and age at onset of Alzheimer's disease. Lancet 348:429–432

Toran-Allerand CD (1991) Organotypic culture of the developing cerebral cortex and hypothalamus: relevance to sexual differentiation. Psychoneuroendocrinology 16:7–24

Toran-Allerand CD, Miranda RC, Bentham WDL, Sohrabji F, Brown TJ, Hochberg RB, MacLusky NJ (1992) Estrogen receptors colocalize with low-affinity nerve growth factor receptors in cholinergic neurons of the basal forebrain. Proc Natl Acad Sci USA 89:4668–4672

van Duijn C, Meijer H, Witteman JCM, Havekes LM, de Knijff P, Van Broeckhoven C, Hofman A (1996) Estrogen, apolipoprotein E and the risk of Alzheimer's disease [abstract]. Neurobiol Aging 16 (suppl): S79–S80

Varney NR, Syrop C, Kubu CS, Struchen M, Hahn S, Franzen K (1993) Neuropsychologic dysfunction in women following leuprolide acetate induction of hypoestrogenism. J Assist Reproduct Genet 10:53–57

Waring SC, Rocca WA, Petersen RC, Kokmen E (1997) Postmenopausal estrogen replacement therapy and Alzheimer's disease: a population-based study in Rochester, Minnesota [abstract]. Neurology 48 (suppl. 2): A79

Wong M, Thompson TL, Moss RL (1996) Nongenomic actions of estrogen in the brain: physiological significance and cellular mechanisms. Crit Rev Neurobiol 10:189–203

Woolley CS, McEwen BS (1992) Estradiol mediates fluctuation in hippocampal synapse density during the estrous cycle in the adult rat. J Neurosci 12:2549–2554

Xu H, Gouras GK, Greenfield JP, Vincent B, Naslund J, Mazzarelli L, Fried G, Javanovic JN, Seeger M, Relkin NR, Liao F, Checler F, Buxbaum JD, Chait BT, Thinakaran G, Sisodia SS, Wang R, Greengard P, Gandy S (1998) Estrogen reduces neuronal generation of Alzheimer β-amyloid peptides. Nature Med 4:447–451

Inflammation, Anti-Inflammatory Drugs and Alzheimer's Disease

*C. H. Kawas**

Summary

Increasing evidence from in vivo and in vitro models suggests that inflammatory processes may contribute to the neuronal dysfunction and degeneration in Alzheimer's disease (AD). Neuritic plaques, a hallmark of AD pathology, have been associated with a host of proteins and acute phase reactants, activated microglia, and complement activation. From these observation, it follows that pharmacological suppression of inflammation may slow the rate of Alzheimer pathology.

Epidemiologic studies and short-term clinical trials, particularly of nonsteroidal anti-inflammatory drugs (NSAIDs), have added support to this hypothesis and suggest a therapeutic potential for anti-inflammatory strategies. Epidemiologic observations have included twin and sibling studies (Breitner et al. 1994, 1995), population based studies (Andersen et al. 1995), and longitudinal studies of patients with AD (Rich et al. 1995). In the Baltimore Longitudinal Study of Aging (Stewart et al. 1997), prospective data suggested that use of NSAIDs for more than two years may reduce the risk of AD by approximately one half. Many studies have been identified by McGeer et al. (1996) as suggesting a protective effect of anti-inflammatory agents, but there have also been numerous studies that do not confirm this effect. Some investigations have even suggested an inverse relationship between the use of NSAIDs and the maintenance of cognitive abilities (Fourrier et al. 1996; Saag et al. 1995).

At present the most commonly used nonsteroidals are nonspecific inhibitors of both isoforms of cycloxygenase (COX 1 and COX 2). Cox 1 is constitutive and most likely mediates the gastric and renal toxicities. COX 2 is inducible and has been noted to be upregulated in neurodegenerative models and in AD. COX 2 might represent an appropriate therapeutic target, and selective COX 2 inhibitors have been developed by industry. They appear to be better tolerated and have good brain penetration. Overall, data from the laboratory as well as epidemiologic studies suggest a potential role for the suppression of inflammation in the treatment and prevention of AD. Confirmation of these findings requires randomized clinical trials, some of which are currently underway.

* Johns Hopkins University School of Medicine, 5501 Hopkins Bayview Circle, Room 1B.82, Baltimore, MD 21224.

R. Mayeux / Y. Christen (Eds.)
Epidemiology of Alzheimer's Disease:
From Gene to Prevention

Introduction

Recent evidence has implicated inflammatory and immune mechanisms in the degenerative process of Alzheimer's Disease (AD). AD lesions are characterized by the presence of numerous inflammatory proteins, including acute phase reactants, inflammatory cytokines (IL-1, IL-6, Tumor Necrosis Factor) and components of the complement cascade, including the Membrane Attack Complex (Itagaki et al. 1994). Nearly all of the inflammatory proteins seen in AD tissue are produced by microglia astrocytes or both (McGeer and McGeer 1995). The presence of activated microglia (macrophages) and reactive astrocytes (Fig. 1) in AD brains led to the hypothesis that anti-inflammatory drugs might be useful to ameliorate the symptoms or even prevent the disorder. Such activated microglia and immune proteins either do not appear in normal adult brain or are markedly upregulated in AD (McGeer and McGeer 1998).

In parallel with these findings from the basic laboratory, some of the most compelling epidemiologic data regarding protection from AD have come from the investigation of anti-inflammatory drugs (particularly NSAIDs) and the risk of AD or rate of disease progression. Although results from these studies have been somewhat mixed, a growing body of epidemiologic evidence suggests that anti-inflammatory drugs may play a role in the prevention and treatment of AD.

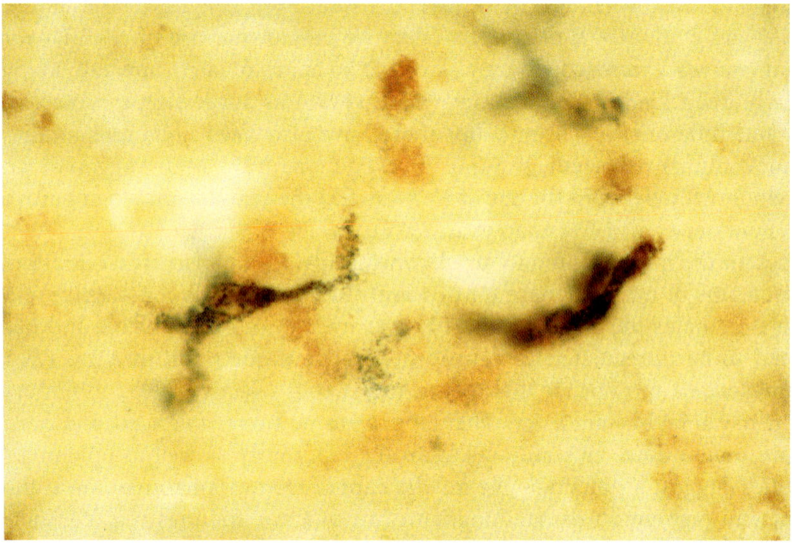

Fig. 1. Immunostaining of the cerebral cortex from an 87-year-old female with autopsy-confirmed AD, demonstrating a senile plaque with activated microglia and IL1-α. Double-labeling immunostaining with HLA-DR antibody for microglia cells (BDHC, blue signal) and an antibody for IL-1α (DAB, brown/gold signal). Magnification 1000 x. Illustration provided by Drs. L. Martin and J. Troncoso, JHMI ADRC

Epidemiologic Studies

Inflammatory Diseases and Risk of AD

Several studies have reported a reduced risk of AD in patients with inflammatory diseases such as arthritis (Jenkinson et al. 1989; Broe et al. 1990; Li et al. 1992; Canadian Study of Health and Aging 1994; McGeer et al. 1990). The question arises whether these subjects have a reduced risk due to their anti-inflammatory treatments or if subjects with a genetic predisposition to inflammatory diseases such as rheumatoid arthritis also have a genetic predisposition toward a reduced risk of AD. In the case of leprosy, studies have suggested that patients who took dapsone, which has anti-inflammatory activity, were less likely to develop AD than those patients who did not receive anti-inflammatory treatment (McGeer et al. 1992).

NSAIDs and Risk of AD

A reduced risk of AD in subjects who use NSAIDs has been reported in several observational studies. Odds ratios and confidence intervals for some of the published studies are summarized in Figure 2 (for an excellent review see McGeer et al. 1996). Most studies that show an effect of NSAIDs on the risk of AD generally

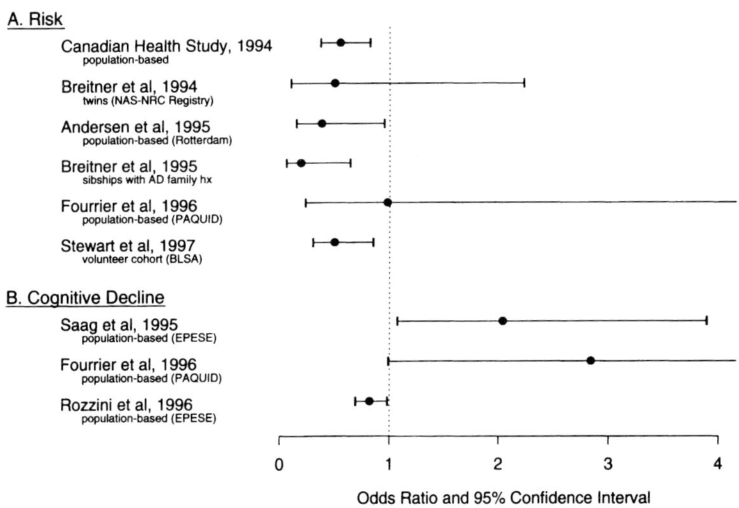

Fig. 2. Epidemiological studies of AD and NSAID use. A) Risk ratio or odds ratio and 95 % confidence interval from studies of AD risk among NSAID users and non-users. Fourrier et al. (1996) report risk of dementia. B) Odds ratio and 95 % confidence interval from studies of cognitive decline among NSAID users and non-users. Saag et al. (1995) report word recall decline over two years, Fourrier et al. (1996) report MMSE decline over two years, and Rozzini et al. (1996) report SPMSQ decline over three years

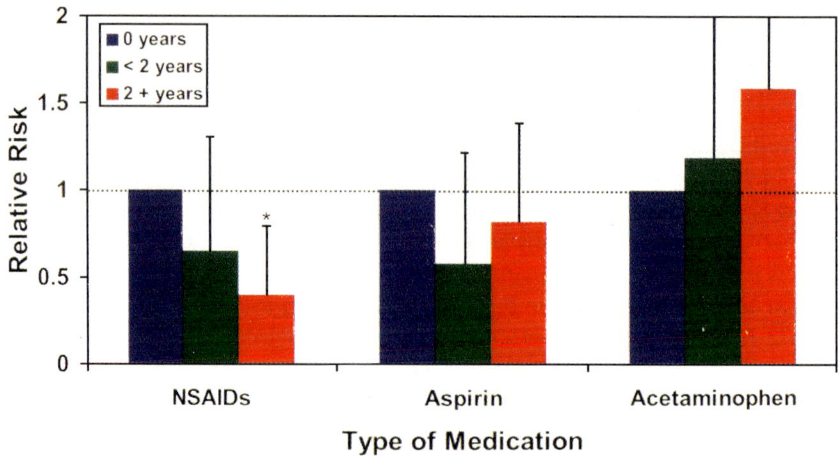

Fig. 3. Relative risk of AD by type and duration of medication use in the BLSA. *$p < 0.05$ from Stewart et al. (1997). Results of Cox proportional hazards regression adjusted for sex and education and using age as the time scale. Study includes 1686 BLSA participants, including 81 AD cases followed up between 1980 and 1995

report about a 50 % reduction in risk. The investigations in Canada (Canadian Study of Health and Aging 1994) and Rotterdam (Andersen et al. 1995) were drawn from population-based samples. Adding additional support, a cohort study in the Baltimore Longitudinal Study of Aging (BLSA/NIA) provided *prospective* data for NSAIDs as a protective factor in AD and, in particular, noted an effect by duration of use. BLSA subjects with two or more years of exposure to NSAIDs had approximately half the risk of AD as subjects who reported less or no exposure (Fig. 3; Stewart et al. 1997).

Risk of Cognitive Decline and NSAIDs

The two studies by Breitner et al. (1994, 1995) were designed to eliminate, or at least minimize, genetic factors. They involve twin pairs or sibships of pedigrees with prominent family histories of AD. When comparing twins discordant for AD by at least three years, the use of steroids appeared to statistically reduce the risk of AD, although much of this exposure consisted of intra-articular injections of steroids for joint disease (Breitner et al. 1994). This finding was not replicated in the subsequent larger studies of sibships with familial AD, but NSAID users in those studies had an odds ratio of 0.19. (95 % CI = 0.058–0.639; Breitner et al. 1995).

Not all investigators, however, have replicated the findings with regards to NSAIDs and the risk of AD (Fourrier et al. 1996). The effect of NSAIDs has also been examined in relationship to cognitive decline in older persons. Data from three communities of the Established Populations for Epidemiologic Studies of the Elderly (EPESE; Rozzini et al. 1996) found Short Portable Mental Status Questionnaire (Pfeiffer 1975) scores after three years to be higher in chronic NSAID users than in non-users. The investigators estimated the magnitude of the effect to be equivalent to a difference in age of onset of 3.5 years. In contrast, investigation of another EPESE sample in rural Iowa (Saag et al. 1995) found high-dose NSAID use to be strongly associated with significant immediate word recall decline. This relationship was only apparent among individuals in the middle two quartiles of recall performance.

Treatment of AD and NSAIDs

In a randomized placebo-controlled trial, Rogers and colleagues noted stable cognitive function over six months in patients treated with indomethacin, whereas significant deterioration was noted in patients on placebo (Rogers et al. 1993). The interpretation of these results was complicated by over one third of the subjects in the drug group dropping out before completion of the six-month trial, largely due to side effects. In an observational analysis, Rich and colleagues noted a slower rate of decline and higher level of functioning in research subjects who were using nonsteroidal anti-inflammatory compounds (Rich et al. 1995).

Broad immuno-suppression is being examined with prednisone treatment in a cohort of patients with mild AD (Multicenter Trial of Prednisone in AD, 1977). This randomized placebo-controlled study of low dose prednisone (20 mg induction with 10 mg Q.D. maintenance) is being conducted by the Alzheimer's Disease Cooperative Study (NIA) and is designed to examine the rate of decline in AD patients followed for 15 months. Results will be available in the near future. This consortium of investigators will also be conducting trials of other anti-inflammatory compounds including hydroxychloroquine and colchicine (Multicenter Trial of Hydroxycloroguine and Colchicine in AD, 1999). Similar trials are already underway in Europe.

Other Anti-inflammatory Treatments

Other anti-inflammatory treatments have been associated with a reduced risk of AD, including prednisone, intra-articular steroids, and ACTH (Breitner et al. 1994). Overall, the number of subjects taking these medications was exceedingly small and it is difficult to draw conclusions from these data. Nonetheless, they lend credence to the hypothesis that suppression of inflammatory mechanisms can be effective in the prevention of AD.

Future Directions

Primary and Secondary Prevention Trials

Although case control and observational studies are crucial for the delineation of potential risk and protective factors, there is no substitute for a randomized clinical trial. The effectiveness of treatments that suppress inflammation must ultimately be determined in randomized clinical trials. To date, no primary prevention trials have been conducted using nonsteroidals in cognitively normal people. Some trials, however, are being conducted in individuals with memory impairment without dementia. These individuals are generally at high risk for developing AD within three to four years (Petersen et al. 1993). In the near future, hopefully, primary prevention trials will be launched.

Selective Cyclooxygenase Inhibition

Glucocorticoids such as prednisone are the most broadly active anti-inflammatory agents in clinical use. Specific actions include suppression of the acute phase response neutrophil adherence and monocyte accumulation as well as inhibition of prostaglandin production (Aisen and Davis 1997). In contrast, nonsteroidal anti-inflammatory drugs do not suppress the acute phase response, but produce inhibition of cyclooxygenase (COX) and antagonism of the effects of interleukin-1. Cyclooxygenase has been identified in two isoforms, COX 1 and COX 2. COX 1 is constitutive and COX 2 is inducible. Both are found in the brain, but COX 1 inhibition largely mediates the effects of gastrointestinal and renal toxicity, whereas COX 2 inhibition suppresses the inflammatory response (Aisen and Davis 1997). Selective COX 2 inhibitors have been developed by industry. For the most part, these compounds have been tested in humans with inflammatory diseases such as arthritis and are well tolerated. They provide a promising approach for future studies in AD.

Impact of Intervention

It is currently estimated that approximately four million people in the United States have AD. The number of individuals with this disorder will quadruple by the middle of the next century if nothing is done to arrest the tide (Brookmeyer et al. 1998). Data from case-control and prospective studies of NSAIDs and AD have shown a reduction of risk consistent with a two- to five-year delay of onset of dementia. The public health impact of delaying AD has been modeled by Brookmeyer and colleagues and is shown in Figure 4. Even modest delays of six months would result in almost half a million fewer people with AD by the middle of the next century. Anti-inflammatory compounds, as well as estrogen and antioxidants, require further investigation of their role in the treatment and prevention of AD. Randomized clinical trials are the crucial next step.

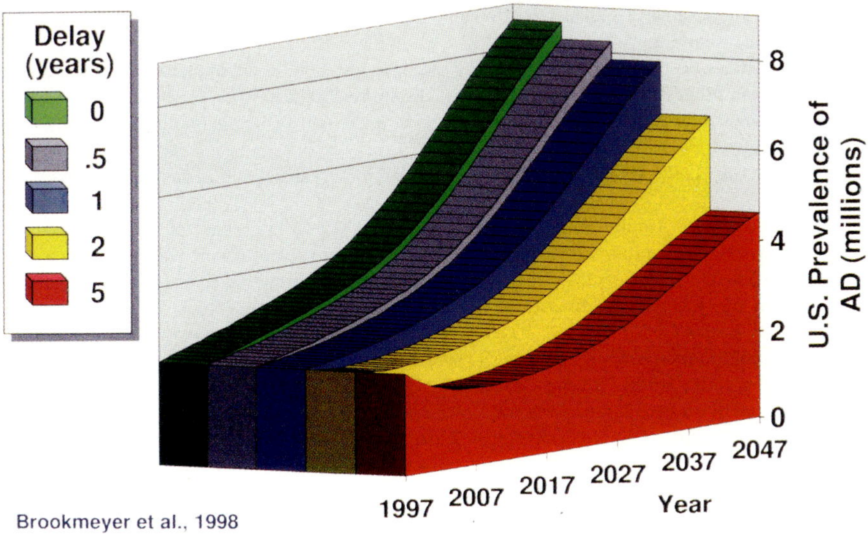

Fig. 4. Potential impact of interventions to delay onset of AD. From Brookmeyer et al. (1998)

References

Aisen PS, Davis KL (1994) Inflammatory mechanisms of Alzheimer's disease: Implications for therapy. Am J Psychiatry 151 (8):1105–1113

Aisen P, Davis K (1997) The search for disease-modifying treatment of Alzheimer's disease. Neurology 48:S35–41

Andersen K, Launer LJ, Ott A, Hoes AW, Breteler MMB, Hofman A (1995) Do nonsteroidal anti-inflammatory drugs decrease the risk of Alzheimer's disease? Neurology 45:1441–1445

Breitner JC, Gau BA, Welsh KA, Plassman BL, McDonald WM, Helms MJ, Anthony JC (1994) Inverse association of anti-inflammatory treatments and Alzheimer's disease: initial results of a co-twin control study. Neurology 44:227–232

Breitner JCS, Welsh KA, Gau BA, McDonald WM, Steffens DC, Saunders AM, Magruder KM, Helms MJ, Plassman BL, Folstein MF, Brandt J, Robinnette CD, Page WF (1995) Alzheimer's Disease in the National Academy of Sciences-National Research Council Registry of Aging Twin Veterans. III. Detection of cases, longitudinal results, and observations on twin concordance. Arch Neurol 52:763–771

Broe GA, Henderson AS, Creasey H, McCusker E, Korten AE, Jorm AF, Longley W, Anthony JC (1990) A case-control study of Alzheimer's disease in Australia. Neurology 40:1698–1707

Brookmeyer R, Gray S, Kawas C (1998) Projections of Alzheimer's disease in the United States and the public health impact of delaying disease onset. Am J Public Health 88:1337–1342

The Canadian Study of Health and Aging (1994): risk factors for Alzheimer's disease in Canada. Neurology 44:2073–2080

Fourrier A LL, Begaud B, Dartigues J-F (1996) Nonsteroidal antiinflammatory drug use and cognitive function in the elderly: Inconclusive results from a population-based cohort study. J Clin Epidemiol 49:1201

Itagaki S, Akiyama H, Saito H, McGeer PL (1994) Ultrastructural localization of complement membrane attack complex (MAC) – like immunoreactivity in brains of patients with Alzheimer's disease. Brain Res 645:78–84

Jenkinson ML, Bliss, MR, Brain AT, Scott DL (1989) Rheumatoid arthritis and senile dementia of the Alzheimer's type. Br J Rheumatol 28:86–88

Li G, Shen YC, Li YT, Chen CH, Zhau YW, Silverman JM (1992) A case-control study of Alzheimer's disease in China. Neurology 42:1481–1488

McGeer PL, McGeer EG (1995) The inflammatory response system of brain: implications for therapy of Alzheimer and other neurodegenerative diseases. Brain Res Brain Res Rev 21:195–218

McGeer E, McGeer P (1998) Inflammation in the brain in Alzheimer's Disease: implications for therapy. NeuroSci News 1:29–35

McGeer PL, McGeer E, Rogers J, Sibley J (1990) Anti-inflammatory drugs and Alzheimer's disease. Lancet 335:1037

McGeer PL, Harada N, Kimura H, McGeer EG, Schulzer M (1992) Prevalence of dementia amongst elderly Japanese with leprosy: apparent effect of chronic drug therapy. Dementia 3:146–149

McGeer PL, Schulzer M, McGeer EG (1996) Arthritis and anti-inflammatory agents as possible protective factors for Alzheimer's disease: A review of 17 epidemiologic studies. Neurology 1996; 47:425–432

Multicenter Trial of Prednisone in Alzheimer's Disease (1997). Project Leader: Paul Aisen, Alzheimer's Disease Cooperative Study, PI: Leon Thal. National Institute on Aging

Multicenter Trial of Hydroxychloroquine and Colchicine in Alzheimer's Disease (1999) Project Leader: Paul Aisen, Alzheimer's Disease Cooperative Study, PI: Leon Thal. National Institute on Aging

Petersen RC, Smith GE, Tangalos EG, Kokmen E, Ivnik RJ (1993) Longitudinal outcome of patients with a mild cognitive impairment. Ann Neurol 34:294–295

Pfeiffer E (1975) A short portable mental status questionnaire for the assessment of organic brain deficit in elederly patients. JAGS 23:433–441

Rich JB, Rasmusson DX, Folstein MF, Carson KA, Kawas CH, Brandt J (1995) Nonsteroidal antiinflammatory drugs in Alzheimer's disease. Neurology 45:51–55

Rogers J, Kirby LC, Hempelman SR, Berry DL, McGeer PL, Kaszniak AW, Zalinski J, Cofield M, Mansukhani L, Willson P, Kogan F (1993) Clinical trial of indomethacin in Alzheimer's disease. Neurology 43:1609–1611

Rozzini R, Ferrucci L, Losonczy K, Havlik RJ, Guralnik JM (1996) Protective effect of chronic NSAID use on cognitive decline in older persons. JAGS 44: 1025–1029

Saag KG, Rubenstein LM, Chrischilles EA, Wallace RB (1995) Nonsteroidal antiinflammatory drugs and cognitive decline in the elderly. J Rheumatol 22:2142–2147

Stewart WF, Kawas C, Corrada M, Metter EJ (1997) Risk of Alzheimer's disease and duration of NSAID use. Neurology 48:626–632

Socio-Demographic Risk Factors for Dementia and Alzheimer's Disease in the Paquid Study

J. F. Dartigues, C. Helmer*, L. Letenneur**

Paquid (Personne Agée QUID) is a French population-based prospective cohort study conducted in the Bordeaux area and specifically designed to study normal and pathological brain aging (Barberger-Gateau et al. 1992). The main objective of Paquid was initially the analysis of the natural history of the cognitive disorders occurring at the very early phase of dementia. However, the baseline data collection and the follow-up of the cohort provided the opportunity to study the relationships between several potential risk factors and the risk of subsequent dementia or Alzheimer's Disease (AD). We will present here some results about these risk factors with special attention to socio-demographic factors such as age, gender, level of education and marital status.

Methods

Sample:

The Paquid research programme was designed to study prospectively a representative random sample of people aged 65 years and over living in Gironde and Dordogne, two administrative areas in southwest France. Subjects were randomly chosen from the electoral rolls of 75 parishes. Three criteria had to be met for subjects to be included in the study: 1) to be at least 65 years of age by December 31, 1987, 2) to be living at home at the time of the initial data collection phase, and 3) to give their informed consent to participate in the study. A three-step random procedure based on the electoral rolls stratified by age, sex and size of the demographic unit was performed. This procedure led to the selection of 5,554 elderly subjects living at home.

* Dartigues JF, INSERM U 330, Université de Bordeaux II, 146 rue Léo Saignat, 33076 Bordeaux Cedex. France. Fax number: (33) 556991360.

R. Mayeux / Y. Christen (Eds.)
Epidemiology of Alzheimer's Disease:
From Gene to Prevention

Data collection

Baseline screening:

Subjects were informed by mail that they had been chosen to participate in a study on the health status and living conditions of people aged 65 years and over. Then subjects were contacted by telephone or visited directly at home if they did not have a telephone. Subjects who agreed to participate were seen by a psychologist specially trained for home interviews. The baseline variables that were registered included socio-demographic factors, social support and network, living conditions and habits, subjective and objective health measures, a comprehensive functional assessment with the Katz scale (Katz et al. 1970) and Lawton and Brody scale (1969), depressive symptomatology measured by the CES-D (Center for Epidemiological Study Depression) scale (Radloff 1977), personal medical history, current symptoms and diseases, and neurosensory deficiencies. A more complete description of the baseline data collected in the Paquid study has been published previously (Barberger-Gateau et al. 1992).

Among the socio-demographic data, we considered age in years, gender and education at four levels: no schooling, primary school level (equivalent of 1 to 5 years of schooling), secondary school level (6 to 12 years of schooling), university level (over 12 years of schooling). The highest diploma attained was also recorded. Marital status was classified into four categories: married or cohabitant, single, widowed and divorced or separated. Evolution of marital status has been considered in the analyses. Married or cohabitant subjects who became widowed during the follow-up were included in the group of married subjects until their widow(er)hood, and in the group of widowed thereafter. Social network was assessed with three variables: subject living alone or not, number of people in the social network and self-perceived satisfaction of this network (very satisfied, satisfied, unsatisfied or very unsatisfied). The number of leisure activities known to be associated with a lower risk of dementia (Fabrigoule et al. 1995) (gardening, travelling and odd job or knitting) was also considered.

Intellectual function was examined through a series of psychometric tests that were among the most sensitive for following cognitive decline in elderly individuals. The test battery included an evaluation of global mental status (Mini Mental State Examination; Folstein et al. 1975), visual memory (Benton's Visual Retention Test; Benton 1965), verbal memory (Wechsler's Paired-Associates; Wechsler 1945), verbal fluency (Isaacs Set Test; Isaacs and Akhtar 1972), visuospatial attention (Zazzo's cancellation test; Zazzo 1964) and simple logical reasoning (Wechsler's Digit Symbol Test; Wechsler 1981).

Diagnosis of Dementia:

After the psychometric evaluation, the psychologists systematically completed a standardized questionnaire designed to obtain the A (memory impairment), B (impairment of at least one other cognitive function) and C (interference with social or professional life) criteria for DSM-III R dementia (APA, 1987). This questionnaire had been previously validated with a good inter-observer reliability between the psychologist and the neurologist on the basis of the DSM-III criteria. In a second stage, subjects who met these first three DSM-III R criteria for dementia were seen by a senior neurologist who confirmed and completed the DSM-III R criteria for dementia and filled in the NINCDS-ADRDA criteria (McKhann et al. 1984) and the Hachinski score (Hachinski et al. 1975) to document the diagnosis of dementia and its aetiology: probable or possible Alzheimer's disease or other type of dementia. When available an informant was consulted by the neurologist.

Follow-Up:

Subjects were re-evaluated, following the same procedure as for the baseline screening, one, three and five years after the initial visit in Gironde and three and five years after the initial visit in Dordogne. At each follow-up assessment, the case finding and the aetiological categorization of incident cases of dementia followed the same procedure as for the baseline screening. Moreover the marital status was collected at each follow-up visit.

Statistical analysis:

Age-specific incidence was estimated using the person-years method (Breslow and Day 1987). The basic method used to estimate age-specific incidence rates is to determine for each individual the amount of observation time contributed to a given age by calendar period category and to sum up those contributions for all cohort members to obtain the total number of person-years in that category. For subjects with more than one follow-up evaluation, person-years were calculated as the time between the baseline visit and the last follow-up examination if the subject remained non-demented. For a demented subject, we considered half of the time between the last visit where the subject was diagnosed demented. Age-specific incidence was computed according to marital status, taking into account the changes with time.

The relative risks (RR) of AD were estimated using a Cox proportional hazards model with delayed entry, in which the time-scale is the age of the subjects. It is now recognized that, in the study of age-associated diseases, the appropriate time-scale for survival models is age rather than time since the baseline survey (Korn et al. 1997; Commenges et at. 1997, 1998). This approach allows one to model directly the risk of dementia according to age, which is no longer included as a covariate. However, as we studied incident cases, the subjects can participate in the analysis only if they did not experience dementia before their inclusion. The sample is left truncated because subjects are observed conditionally because they did not develop a dementia before entering the cohort. To deal with the left truncation, we used a Cox model with delayed entry, where a subject is considered to be at risk of dementia between the age at entry to the cohort and the age of censorship or the age at onset of the disease (Commenges et al. 1998). Marital status was considered as a time-dependent covariate.

Results and Discussion

Of the 5,554 contacted subjects, a total of 3,777 (68 %) agreed to participate in the study. Non-responders did not differ from responders in age, gender or educational level (Dartigues et al. 1991). Among the 3,675 initially non-demented subjects of the cohort, 2,133 (58 %) were women and 1,822 subjects (49.6 %) were older than 74. The baseline marital status was distributed as followed: 2,106 married or cohabitant (57.3 %), 1287 widowed (35 %), 179 singles (4.9 %) and 103 divorced or separated (2.8 %).

Of the 3,675 subjects, 794 (21.6 %) did not participate in the follow-up because they died (n = 365; 9.9 %) or because they were lost to follow-up or refused the follow-up screenings (n = 429; 11.7 %). At least one complete follow-up evaluation was performed on 2,881 (78.4 %). During the five years of follow-up, 222 initially married or cohabitant subjects became widowed (10.5 %).

One hundred and ninety subjects developed an incident dementia, of whom 140 were classified as incident cases of AD and 50 as other type of dementia. Overall incidences of dementia and AD were estimated as 1.59 person-years and 1.17 person-years, respectively. The global incidence of dementia was estimated as 1.3 per 100 person-years in men and 1.8 in women (0.8 and 1.4 for AD, respectively). The incidence of AD was higher in men before 80 years and higher in women after 80 years. The relative risk (RR) of a woman developing AD was then estimated to be 0.83 at age 75 and 1.72 at age 85.

We studied the risk of AD in subjects with no schooling and in subjects with a primary school level, taking subjects with a secondary or university level as the reference. We found a higher risk of developing AD in subjects with no schooling (RR = 1.93, p = 0.04) and in subjects who attained a primary school level (RR = 1.49, p = 0.02). But the categorisation does not seem to be the best one. The best prediction of AD was obtained with the cut-off primary school level not validated by a diploma (in French, "certificat d'étude primaire") versus higher education (RR = 1.83, p = 0.00001). The relative risk of gender and education were unchanged when gender was adjusted for education. Thus a confounding effect of education seems unlikely to explain the risk of dementia or AD observed in women.

Taking the married subjects as the reference group, the risk of dementia was significantly greater in singles (RR = 1.77, 95 % CI = 1.05–3.00). The risk of dementia did not changed for widowed or divorced subjects. The same trends were observed for the risk of AD, but the RR was greater for singles (RR = 2.39, 95 % CI = 1.34–4.25). On the contrary, the RR of non-AD dementia for singles was lower than one and not significantly different from married subjects.

After adjustment for possible confounding factors such as gender, educational level, principal occupation during life and wine consumption, the relationship between marital status and risk of AD remained unchanged. In addition, the introduction of the marital status in the model did not change the significant relationship between education or wine consumption and the risk of AD. Widowed subjects have almost the same risk as married subjects.

In conclusion, socio-demographic factors such as gender, educational level and marital status seem to be major risk factors of AD in old age with a similar magnitude as genetic factors like apoE4 allele. For instance, the population-based attributable risk of AD related to low education could be estimated at 18.9 %. These findings need of course to be confirmed and explained by further studies and could be part of the detection of high risk subjects for AD.

Acknowledgements

This study was supported by grants from the Fondation de France, Novartis Laboratories, Axa Insurance Group, Conseil Général de la Gironde, Conseil Générale de la Dordogne, Ministère de la Recherche et de la Technologie, Caisse Nationale d'Assurance Maladie, Caisse Primaire d'Assurance Maladie de Dordogne, Mutualité Sociale Agricole de Gironde et Dordogne, Mutuelle Générale de l'Education Nationale, Conseil Régional d'Aquitaine, Société Pechiney, Société BSN, 2010 Media, Caisse de Retraite Interentreprise, Capimmec, Institut du Cerveau, Direction Régionale des Affaires Sanitaires et Sociales d'Aquitaine.

References

APA (1987) Diagnostic and statistical manual of mental disorders, Edition III Revised (DSM-III R). Washington DC, American Psychiatric Association

Barberger-Gateau P, Chaslerie A, Dartigues JF, Commenges D, Gagnon M, Salamon R (1992) Health measures correlates in a French elderly population: the Paquid study. J Gerontol 47:S88–S95

Benton A (1965) Manuel pour l'application du test de rétention visuelle. Applications cliniques et expérimentales. Paris, Centre de Psychologie Appliquée

Breslow N, Day N (1987) Statistical method in cancer research. Vol. 2. Lyon, IARC Scientific Publications n° 82, WHO

Commenges D, Letenneur L, Joly P (1997) Re: „Serum transferrin saturation, stroke incidence, and mortality in women and men. The NHANES I Epidemiologic Follow-up Study." Am J Epidemiol 146:683–684

Commenges D, Letenneur L, Joly P, Alioum A, Dartigues JF (1998) Modelling age-specific risk: application to dementia. Stat Med 17:1973–1988

Dartigues, JF, Gagnon M, Michel P, Letenneur L, Commenges D, Barberger-Gateau P, Auriacombe S, Rigal B, Bedry R, Alperovitch A, Orgogozo JM, Henry P, Loiseau P, Salamon R (1991) Le programme de recherche Paquid sur l'épidémiologie de la démence. Méthodologie et résultats initiaux. Rev Neurol (French) 147:225–230

Fabrigoule C, Letenneur L, Dartigues JF, Zarrouk M, Commenges D, Barberger-Gateau P (1995) Social and leisures activities and risk of dementia: a prospective longitudinal study. J Am Geriatr Soc 43:485–490

Folstein MF, Folstein SE, McHugh PR (1975) Mini-Mental State. A practical method for grading the cognitive state of patients for the clinicians. J Psychiatr Res 12:189–198

Hachinski VC, Iliff LD, Zilhka F, Du Boulay GH, McAllister VL, Marshall J, Russell RWR, Symon L (1975) Cerebral blood flow in dementia. Arch Neurol 32:632–637

Isaacs B, Akhtar A (1972) The set test: a rapid test of mental function in old people. Age Aging 1:222–226

Katz S, Downs T, Cash H, Grotz R (1970) Progress in development of the index of A.D.L. Gerontologist 10:20–30

Korn EL, Graubard BI, Midthune D (1997) Time-to-event analysis of longitudinal follow-up of a survey: choice of the time-scale. Am J Epidemiol 145:72–80

Lawton M, Brody E (1969) Assessment of older people: self-maintaining and instrumental activities of daily living. Gerontologist 9:179–186

McKhann G, Drachman D, Folstein M, Katzman R, Price D, Stadlan EM (1984) Clinical diagnosis of Alzheimer's disease: report of the NINCDS-ADRDA work group under the auspices of the Department of Health and Human Services task force on Alzheimer's disease. Neurology 34:939–944

Radloff LS (1977) The CES-D scale: a self-report depression scale for research in the general population. Appl Psychol Meas 1:385–401

Wechsler D (1945) A standardized memory scale for clinical use. J Psychol 19:87–95

Wechsler D (1981) Wechsler Adult Intelligence Scale Manual. New York Psychological Corp

Zazzo R (1964) Test des deux barrages. Actualités pédagogiques et psychologiques. Neuchâtel, Delachaux et Niestlé

Vascular Disease and Vascular Risk Factors and Dementia

M. M. B. Breteler[1], A. Ott, MD[1, 2], A. Hofman[1]

Introduction

In recent years evidence has increased that vascular disease is associated with cognitive impairment and dementia (Breteler et al. 1994; Hofman et al. 1997). Moreover, the presence of cerebrovascular disease may intensify the presence and severity of the clinical symptoms of Alzheimer's disease (Snowdon et al. 1997).

In this paper, current knowledge about the relation between vascular factors and dementia will be reviewed. We will focus on established risk factors for vascular disease, including age and gender, socio-economic status, diabetes, cholesterol, cigarette smoking and alcohol use, and on indicators of vascular disease, including atherosclerosis and atrial fibrillation.

Established Vascular Risk Factors

Age and Gender

Age is by far the most important risk factor for dementia. The incidence of dementia and Alzheimer's disease increases exponentially with age (Breteler et al. 1992; van Duijn 1996; Ott et al. 1998 a). Based on several recent prospective population-based studies, the incidence increases roughly from 1 per 1000 person-years in 65 years olds, and 1 per 100 person-years in 75 years olds, to almost 1 per 10 person-years in subjects above age 90.

Reliable age- and gender-specific estimates of the incidence of dementia exist only for subjects over the age of 60. Gender-specific incidence rates are quite sim-

[1] Department of Epidemiology & Biostatistics, Erasmus University Medical School, PO Box 1738, 3000 DR Rotterdam, The Netherlands.
[2] Department of Medical Microbiology, University Hospital Rotterdam, Dr. Molewaterplein 40, 3015 GD Rotterdam, The Netherlands.
Correspondence to:
Monique M. B. Breteler, MD, PhD, Department of Epidemiology & Biostatistics, Erasmus University Medical School, PO Box 1738, 3000 DR Rotterdam, The Netherlands, tel +31 10 408 7489, fax +31 10 436 5933, email breteler@epib.fgg.eur.nl.

R. Mayeux / Y. Christen (Eds.)
Epidemiology of Alzheimer's Disease:
From Gene to Prevention

ilar until the age of 85, after which incidence rates seem higher for women than for men (Ott et al. 1998 a; Fratiglioni et al. 1997).

Socio-Economic Status

Various studies have shown a relation between low socio-economic status and vascular disease. However, different indicators of socio-economic status may yield different results. For example, in a Danish study, household income was associated with the risk of stroke but years of education was not (Boysen et al. 1988). Many studies have examined the relation between educational background and dementia or Alzheimer's disease and suggested that higher educational levels were protective against dementia (Katzman 1993; Ott et al. 1995). However, most of these studies were cross-sectional and had ample potential for bias. Indeed, population-based studies of incident cases yielded no or smaller effects of education on risk of dementia or Alzheimer's disease (Beard et al. 1992; Cobb et al. 1995; Ott 1997). Other indicators of socio-economic status have not been reported in relation to dementia.

Diabetes mellitus

Some older cross-sectional case-control studies showed diabetes mellitus to be positively associated with vascular dementia but inversely associated with Alzheimer's disease (Bucht et al. 1983; Landin et al. 1993; Mortel et al. 1993; Nielson et al. 1996; Wolf-Klein et al. 1998). However, these studies were based on selected patients and controls, the presence of diabetes mellitus was assessed from medical records and not actually screened for, and subjects with any indication of vascular disease were often rigorously excluded from the Alzheimer patient series. In contrast, a cross-sectional analysis based on the Rotterdam Study, a population-based cohort study of subjects aged 55 and over, showed that subjects with diabetes mellitus had dementia more often than those without diabetes mellitus (odds ratio 1.3; 95 % CI 1.0–1.9), in particular subjects who needed insulin treatment (odds ratio 3.2; 95 % CI 1.4–7.5). The relation was strongest with vascular dementia but was also found for Alzheimer's disease (Ott et al. 1996). Recently, this positive association between diabetes mellitus and Alzheimer's disease was confirmed in several longitudinal studies. A register-based retrospective cohort study from Rochester, MN, reported an increased risk for dementia and its subtype Alzheimer's disease (RR 1.7; 95 % CI 1.3–2.1; Leibson et al. 1997). In a prospective population-based study among 828 elderly Japanese, diabetics had a more than two-fold increased risk of Alzheimer's disease (RR 2.2; 95 % CI 1.0–4.9; Yoshitake et al. 1995). Similarly, among 6370 subjects of the Rotterdam Study who were followed prospectively, a relative risk of Alzheimer's disease of 1.9 (95 % CI 1.2–3.1) was found. The risk for Alzheimer's disease was highest among subjects who were treated with insulin (RR 4.3; 95 % CI 1.7–10.5; Ott 1997).

The mechanism through which diabetes mellitus increases the risk of cerebrovascular disease is not entirely clear. Evidently, diabetes is associated with micro- and macrovascular changes. However, the risk of stroke is increased independently from other vascular risk factors, and there might also be a direct effect of glucose on the cerebral vasculature. Intensive treatment of diabetes and good metabolic control reduce the risk of stroke (DCCT Research Group 1993; Kuusisto et al. 1994). In Alzheimer's disease, hyperglycemia may potentiate the deleterious effect of other pathological processes taking place, such as amyloid deposition (Messier and Gagnon 1996). On the other hand, hypoglycemia has a direct effect on cerebral functioning, and the resulting damage may accumulate with the number of hypoglycemic periods.

Cholesterol

An elevated level of plasma cholesterol is a strong risk factor for coronary vascular disease. The relation between cholesterol and cerebrovascular disease remains controversial (Prospective Studies Cooperation 1995; Gorelick et al. 1997; Wolf et al. 1992). There is some evidence that a high cholesterol level may increase the risk of stroke in younger subjects but is not related to the occurrence of stroke among elderly subjects. There have been few reports in the literature on the relation between plasma cholesterol levels and Alzheimer's disease. A small hospital-based case-control study suggested that Alzheimer patients have higher mean total cholesterol levels than controls (Giubilei et al. 1990) and, because of the relation between APOE genotype and cholesterol level, the effect of the APOE genotype might depend on cholesterol levels (Jarvik et al. 1995). However, the bulk of the evidence does not point to an important relation between cholesterol level and Alzheimer's disease.

Smoking

Smoking undoubtedly increases the risk of stroke (Bartecchi et al. 1994; Shinton and Beevers 1989). The relation between smoking and Alzheimer's disease is much disputed. A meta-analysis on case-control studies conducted before 1990 suggested an inverse association between Alzheimer's disease and history of smoking (Graves et al. 1991). Studies conducted since then showed no relation (Yoshitake et al. 1995; Canadian Study of Health and Aging 1994; Forster et al. 1995; Hebert et al. 1992), an inverse relation (Brenner et al. 1993; Letenneur et al. 1994), or a positive relation (Prince et al. 1994). There are some biologically plausible explanations for a protective effect of smoking on Alzheimer's disease, including a memory and cognition enhancing effect of nicotine, possibly through increasing the density of nicotine receptors of facilitating the release of acetylcholine (Newhouse et al. 1994; Nitta et al. 1994). However, one should consider that some of the findings in previous studies may have resulted from bias (Riggs 1993). Most previous studies were cross-sectional and based on prevalent cases.

A recent prospective analysis on incident cases of the Rotterdam Study showed that people who smoked cigarettes had a more than two-fold increased risk of Alzheimer's disease (Ott et al. 1998b). Besides bias, an explanation for the discrepant findings may be that some of the earlier studies that showed a protective effect of smoking included younger cases. It is conceivable that the relation between smoking and Alzheimer's disease is age-dependent, for example because of different genetic susceptibility. Some support for this hypothesis comes from the observation among early-onset patients that the inverse association between smoking and Alzheimer's disease was limited to carriers of the apolipoprotein E4 allele (van Duijn et al. 1995). Smoking may exert different and opposite effects on the risk of Alzheimer's disease, being generally harmful through, for example, a vascular mechanism, but also partly beneficial in specific individuals, especially in those who carry an apolipoprotein E4 allele. This hypothesis may be supported by the observation that, in Alzheimer patients, carriers of apolipoprotein E4 have fewer nicotinic receptor binding sites and decreased activity of choline acetyltransferase, as compared to non-carriers of this allele (Poirier et al. 1995). In the Rotterdam Study the elevated relative risk was particularly present for smokers without the apolipoprotein E4 allele, a finding that also in line with this hypothesis (Ott et al. 1998b).

Alcohol

The relation between alcohol intake and the risk of any cerebrovascular disease follows a J-shape. Moderate alcohol consumption decreases the risk of ischemic stroke (Jamrozik et al. 1994; Stampfer et al. 1988). However, with increasing alcohol intake the risk of stroke gradually increases, in particular the risk of hemorrhagic stroke. Most studies reported no evidence for an altered risk of Alzheimer's disease in people with moderate alcohol intake (Graves et al. 1991; Canadian Study of Health and Aging 1994; Brenner et al. 1993), but alcohol abuse has been reported to significantly increase the risk of dementia or Alzheimer's disease (Fratiglioni et al. 1993; Saunders et al. 1991). Recently, the Paquid study, a population-based prospective study in Gironde, France, reported a protective effect from alcohol consumption on the risk of dementia (Orgogozo et al. 1997). Preliminary data from the Rotterdam Study seem to confirm this finding (Breteler et al. 1997).

Indicators of Vascular Disease

Atherosclerosis

Prior cardiovascular events and existing atherosclerosis are well-recognized risk factors for cerebrovascular events (Kannel et al. 1983; Norris et al. 1991). Clinical (cardio)vascular disease has hardly been studied in relation to Alzheimer's disease. Because of the diagnostic criteria for Alzheimer's disease, patients with overt vascular disease are less likely to be diagnosed as Alzheimer patients (Breteler et al. 1992). In a cross-sectional analysis from the Rotterdam Study, indicators of atherosclerosis of the carotid arteries (wall thickness and plaques as measured by ultra-sonography) and the presence of atherosclerosis of the large vessels of the legs (assessed by the ratio of the ankle-to-brachial systolic blood pressure) were associated with Alzheimer's disease. The prevalence of Alzheimer's disease increased with the degree of atherosclerosis. The odds ratio for Alzheimer's disease in those with severe atherosclerosis was 3.0 (95% CI 1.5–6.0) as compared to those without atherosclerosis. A strong interaction between APOE4 and atherosclerosis was observed. Subjects with at least one APOE4 allele and severe atherosclerosis had a nearly 20-fold increased risk for Alzheimer's disease (Hofman et al. 1997).

Atrial fibrillation

Atrial fibrillation is a common finding in the elderly and an important risk factor for cerebral infarctions, which often remain clinically silent (Ezekowitz et al. 1995; Peterson 1990). Cardiac dysrythmias have long been suspected to aggravate or precipitate dementia (Cardiogenic Dementia 1977), yet studies on cognitive performance or risk of dementia in patients with atrial fibrillation are rare. In the Rotterdam Study, atrial fibrillation as assessed in standard 12-lead ECGs was significantly more frequent among subjects with dementia (age and gender adjusted odds ratio 2.3; 95% CI 1.4–3.7) than in those without. The relation was slightly stronger for subjects with Alzheimer's disease than for subjects with vascular dementia and could not be explained by a history of stroke. Most likely the association is due to the hypercoagulable state in subjects with atrial fibrillation which results in an increased risk of cerebral thromboembolism. The associations were stronger in women than in men (age adjusted odds ratio for dementia 3.1 (95% CI 1.7–5.5) and 1.3 (95% CI 0.5–3.1), respectively; Ott et al. 1997). Interestingly, two population-based prospective studies on atrial fibrillation and stroke showed similar gender differences; in both the Copenhagen City Heart Study and the Framingham Study women with atrial fibrillation had higher relative risks of stroke than men (Boysen et al. 1988; Wolf et al. 1991). These gender differences may be due to different etiologies underlying atrial fibrillation in men and women.

Conclusion

Alzheimer's disease is a common disorder in older age. Notwithstanding much research effort, its etiology is still largely unknown. Etiological research in Alzheimer's disease that also focusses on vascular risk factors is relatively new, and available evidence is still limited. However, many of the classical risk factors for vascular disease, as well as markers of atherosclerosis, seem to increase the risk for both dementia and its subtype, Alzheimer's disease. Based on existing epidemiological evidence it is impossible to distinguish what underlies these associations. It may be that vascular disease and Alzheimer's disease have, to some extent, a shared etiology, and that the risk factors that they have in common increase the risk of both disorders independently. Another possibility is that vascular disease is involved in the etiology of Alzheimer's disease. Finally, what is considered Alzheimer's disease on clinical grounds may actually be a mixed bag of dementing syndromes due to cerebrovascular pathology, Alzheimer pathology, or a combination of the two. And the association may be with the vascular component of the dementia syndromes rather than with the Alzheimer pathology. Further research is required to unravel which and how vascular risk factors contribute to dementia.

Acknowledgments

The research of Dr. Monique M. B. Breteler has been made possible by a fellowship from the Royal Netherlands Academy of Arts and Sciences.

References

Bartecchi CE, MacKenzie TD, Schrier RW (1994) The human costs of tobacco use (1), N Engl J Med 330:907–912

Beard CM, Kokmen E, Offord KP, Kurland LT (1992) Lack of association between Alzheimer's disease and education, occupation, marital status, or living arrangement. Neurology 42:2063–2068

Boysen G, Nyboe J, Appleyard M, Sørensen PS, Boas J, Somnier F, Jensen G, Schnohr P (1988) Stroke incidence and risk factors for stroke in Copenhagen, Denmark. Stroke 19:1345–1353

Brenner DE, Kukull WA, van Belle G, Bowen JD, McCormick WC, Teri L, Larson EB (1993) Relationship between cigarette smoking and Alzheimer's disease in a population-based case-control study. Neurology 43:293–300

Breteler MMB, Claus JJ, Launer LJ, van Duijn CM, Hofman A (1992) Epidemiology of Alzheimer's disease. Epidemiol Rev 14:59–82

Breteler MMB, Claus JJ, Grobbee DE, Hofman A (1994) Cardiovascular disease and the distribution of cognitive function in an elderly population. The Rotterdam Study. BMJ 308:1604–1608

Breteler MMB, Mehta K, Ott A, Witteman JCM, Hofman A (1997) Alcohol consumption and dementia. The Rotterdam Study. (Abstract) J Neurol 244 (Suppl 3):S47

Bucht G, Adolfsson R, Lithner R, Winblad B (1983) Changes in blood glucose and insulin secretion in patients with senile dementia of Alzheimer type. Acta Med Scand 213:387–392

Canadian Study of Health and Aging (1994) Risk factors for Alzheimer's disease in Canada. Neurology 44:2073–2080

Cardiogenic Dementia (1977) Lancet i, 27–28

Cobb JL, Wolf PA, Au R, White R, D'Agostino RB (1995) The effect of education on the incidence of dementia and Alzheimer's disease in the Framingham Study. Neurology 45:1707–1712

DCCT Research Group (1993) The Effect of intensive treatment of diabetes on the development and progression of long-term complications in insulin dependent diabetes mellitus. N Engl J Med 329:977–986

Ezekowitz MD, James KE, Nazarian SM, Davenpoort J, Broderick JP, Gupta SR, Thadani V, Meyer ML, Bridgers SL (1995) Silent cerebral infarction in patients with nonrheumatic atrial fibrillation. Circulation 92:2178–2182

Forster DP, Newens AJ, Kay DW, Edwardson JA (1995) Risk factors in clinically diagnosed presenile dementia of the Alzheimer type: a case-control study in northern England. J Epidemiol Comm Health 49:253–258

Fratiglioni L, Ahlbom A, Viitanen M, Winblad B (1993) Risk factors for late-onset Alzheimer's disease: a population-based, case-control study. Ann Neurol 33:258–266

Fratiglioni L, Viitanen M, von Strauss E, Tontodonati V, Herlitz A, Winblad B (1997) Very old women at highest risk of dementia and Alzheimer's disease: incidence data from the Kungsholmen Project, Stockholm. Neurology 48:132–138

Giubilei F, D Antona R, Antonini R, Lenzi GL, Ricci G, Fieschi C (1990) Serum lipoprotein pattern variations in dementia and ischemic stroke. Acta Neurol Scand 81(1): 84–86

Gorelick PB, Schneck M, Berglund LF, Feinberg W, Goldstone J (1997) Status of lipids as a risk factor for stroke. Neuroepidemiology 16:107–115

Graves AB, van Duijn CM, Chandra V, Fratiglioni L, Heyman A, Jorm AF, Kokmen E, Kondo K, Mortimer JA, Rocca WA, Shalat SL, Soininen H, Hofman A (1991) Alcohol and tobacco consumption as risk factors of Alzheimer's disease: a collaborative re-analysis of case-control studies. EURODEM Risk Factors Research Group. Int J Epidemiol 20 (Suppl 2): S48–57

Hebert LE, Scherr PA, Beckett LA, Funkenstein HH, Albert MS, Chown MJ, Evans DA (1992) Relation of smoking and alcohol consumption to incident Alzheimer's disease. Am J Epidemiol 135:347–355

Hofman A, Ott A, Breteler MMB, Bots ML, Slooter AJC, van Harskamp F, van Duijn CM, Van Broeckhoven C, Grobbee DE (1997) Atherosclerosis, apolopoprotein-E and the prevalence of dementia and Alzheimer's disease in the Rotterdam Study. Lancet 349:151–154

Jamrozik K, Phil D, Broadhurst J, Anderson CS, Stewart-Wynne E (1994) The role of lifestyle factors in the etiology of stroke. A population-based case-control study in Perth, Western Australia. Stroke 25:51–59

Jarvik GP, Wijsman EM, Kukull WA, Schellenberg GD, Yu C, Larson EB (1995) Interactions of apolipoprotein E genotype, total cholesterol level, age, and sex in prediction of Alzheimer's disease: a case-control study. Neurology 45:1092–1096

Kannel WB, Wolf PA, Verter J (1983) Manifestation of coronary disease predisposing to stroke. The Framingham Study. JAMA 250:2942–2946

Katzman R (1993) Education and the prevalence of dementia and Alzheimer's disease. Neurology 43:13–20

Kuusisto J, Mykkänen L, Pyörälä K, Laaks OM (1994) Non insulin dependent diabetes and its metabolic control are important predictors of stroke in elderly subjects. Stroke 25:1157–1164

Landin K, Blennow K, Wallin A, Gottfries CG (1993) Low blood pressure and blood glucose levels in Alzheimer's disease. Evidence for a hypometabolic disorder? J Intern Med 233:357–363

Leibson CL, Rocca WA, Hanson VA, Cha R, Kokmen E, O'Brian PC, Palumbo PJ (1997) Risk of dementia among persons with diabetes mellitus: A population-based cohort study. Am J Epidemiol 145:301–308

Letenneur L, Dartigues JF, Commenges D, Burberger-Gateau P, Tessier JF, Orgogozo JM (1994) Tobacco consumption and cognitive impairment in elderly people. A population-based study. Ann Epidemiol 4:449–454

Messier C, Gagnon M (1996) Glucose regulation and cognitive functions: relation to Alzheimer's disease and diabetes. Behav Brain Res 75:1–11

Mortel KF, Wood S, Pavol MA, Meyer JS, Rexer JL (1993) Analysis of familial and individual risk factors among patients with ischemic vascular dementia and Alzheimer's disease. Angiology 44:599–605

Newhouse PA, Potter A, Corwin J, Lenox R (1994) Age-related effects of the nicotinic antagonist mecamylamine on cognition and behavior. Neuropsychopharmacology 10:93–107

Nielson KA, Nolan JH, Brechtold NC, Sandman CA, Mulnard RA, Cotman CW (1996) Apolopoprotein-E genotyping of diabetic dementia patients: is diabeters rare in Alzheimer's disease? J Am Geriatr Soc 44:897–904

Nitta A, Katono Y, Itoh A, Hasegawa T, Nabeshima T (1994) Nicotine reverses scopolamine-induced impairment of performance in passive avoidance task in rats through its action on the dopaminergic neuronal system. Pharmacol Biochem Behav 49:807–812

Norris JW, Zhu CZ, Bornstein NM, Chambers BR (1991) Vascular risk of asymptomatic carotid stenosis. Stroke 22:1485–1490

Orgogozo JM, Dartigues JF, Lafont S, Letenneur L, Commenges D, Salamon R, Renaud S, Breteler MMB (1997) Wine consumption and dementia in the elderly: a prospective community study in the Bordeaux area. Rev Neurol (Paris) 153:185–192

Ott A (1997) Risk of dementia: the Rotterdam study. (Thesis) Erasmus University, Rotterdam pp 49–61

Ott A, Breteler MMB, van Harskamp F, Claus JJ, van der Cammen TJM, Grobbee DE, Hofman A (1995) Prevalence of Alzheimer's disease and vascular dementia: association with education. The Rotterdam Study. BMJ 310:970–973

Ott A, Stolk RP, Hofman A, Van Harskamp F, Grobbee DE, Breteler MMB (1996) Association of diabetes mellitus and dementia: The Rotterdam study. Diabetologia 39:1392–1397

Ott A, Breteler MMB, De Bruyne MC, Van Harskamp F, Grobbee DE, Hofman A (1997) Atrial fibrillation and dementia in a population-based study. The Rotterdam Study. Stroke 28:316–321

Ott A, Breteler MMB, Van Harskamp F, Stijnen T, Hofman A (1998 a) The incidence and risk of dementia. The Rotterdam Study. Am J Epidemiol 147:574–580

Ott A, Slooter AJC, Hofman A, Van Harskamp F, Witteman JCM, Van Broeckhoven C, Van Duijn CM, Breteler MMB (1998 b) Smoking and the risk of dementia and Alzheimer's disease in a population-based cohort study: the Rotterdam Study. Lancet 1998; 351:1840–1843

Petersen P (1990) Thromboembolie complications in atrial fibrillation. Stroke 21:4–13

Poirier J, Delisle M-C, Quirion R, Aubert I, Falow M, Lahir D, Hui S, Betrand P, Nalbantoglu J, Gilfix BM, Gauthier S (1995) Apolipoprotein E4 allele as a precictor of cholinergic deficits and treatment outcome in Alzheimer disease. Proc Natl Acad Sci USA 92:12260–12264

Prince M, Cullen M, Mann A (1994) Risk factors for Alzheimer's disease and dementia: A case-control study based on the MRC elderly hypertension trial. Neurology 44:97–104

Prospective Studies Collaboration (1995) Cholesterol, diastolic blood pressure, and stroke: 13,000 strokers in 450,000 people in 45 prospective cohorts. Lancet 346:1647–1653

Riggs JE (1993) Smoking and Alzheimer's disease: protective effect or differential survival bias? Lancet 342:793–794

Saunders PA, Copeland JR, Dewey ME, Davidson IA, McWilliam C, Sharma V, Sullivan C (1991) Heavy drinking as a risk factor for depression and dementia in elderly men. Finding from the Liverpool longitudinal study. Br J Psychiat 159:213–216

Shinton R, Beevers G (1989) Meta-analysis of the relation between cigarette smoking and stroke. BMJ 298:789–794

Snowdon DA, Greiner LH, Mortimer JA, Riley KP, Greiner PA, Markesbery WR (1997) Brain infarction and the clinical expression of Alzheimer disease. The Nun Study. JAMA 277:813–817

Stampfer MJ, Colditz GA, Willett WC, Speizer FE, Hennekens CH (1988) A prospective study of moderate alcohol consumption and the risk of coronary disease and stroke in women. N Engl J Med 319:267–273

Van Duijn CM (1996) Epidemiology of the dementias: recent developments and new approaches. J Neurol Neurosurg Psychiat 60:478–488

Van Duijn CM, Havekes LM, Van Broeckhoven C, De Knijff P, Hofman A (1995) Apolipoprotein E genotype and association between smoking and early onset Alzheimer's disease. Brit Med J 310:627–631

Wolf PA, D'Agostino RB, Belanger AJ, Kannel WB (1991) Probability of stroke; a risk profile from the Framingham Study. Stoke 22:312–318

Wolf PA, Cobb JL, D Agostino RB (1992) Epidemiology of stroke. In: Barnett HJM, Mohr JP, Stein BM et al. (eds.) Stroke: pathophysiology, diagnosis and management. Second edition. New York, Churchill-Livingstone

Wolf-Klein GP, Siverstone FA, Brod MS, Levy A, Foley CJ, Termotto V, Breuer J (1988) Are Alzheimer patients healthier? J Am Geriatr Soc 36:219–224

Yoshitake T, Kiyohara Y, Kato I, Ohmura T, Iwamoto H, Nakayama K, Ohmori S, Nomiyama K, Kawano H, Ueda K, Sueishi K, Tsuneyeshi M, Fujishima M (1995) Incidence and risk factors of vascular dementia and Alzheimer's disease in a defined elderly Japanese population: the Hisayama Study. Neurology 45:1161–1168

Alzheimer's Disease: A Review of Cross Cultural Studies

*H. C. Hendrie**

Introduction

The dementing disorders affect approximately 5 to 11% of the community-dwelling population aged 65 years and over in Western societies, with the prevalence rates approximately doubling every five years after age 65 and rising to more than 30% in patients 85 years of age and over (Rocca et al. 1986; Torm et al. 1987; Evans et al. 1989; Henderson 1988). If milder forms of the syndrome are included, an additional 10% or more of the elderly population may be affected (Hendrie 1998). Approximately half or more of all nursing home residents have dementia (Class et al. 1996). In most studies, Alzheimer's disease (AD) accounts for approximately two-thirds of all cases of dementia (Hendrie 1998). It has been estimated that the cost to the United States for dementia in 1991 was $67 billion (Ernst and Hay 1996). The direct expenditures in the United Kingdom have been estimated at £738 million (Smith et al. 1995). These costs ignore the enormous impact, both social and economic, on care givers. Dementia, therefore, represents a major public health problem for Western society and one that is only likely to increase over the next several decades, given the current demographic trends. The impact of the dementing disorders has been less well studied in disadvantaged minority groups in countries such as the United States and in developing countries, where the emphasis on healthcare has been focused on children and women of childbearing age. When it is considered, however, that in the United States the so-called minority groups will represent the majority of the population by the mid-twenty-first century, and that already more than half of the elderly in the world live in developing countries where health care resources are less available than in Western countries, studies in these populations become vital (Osuntokun et al. 1992).

Comparative cross-cultureal and trans-national studies of dementia, particularly those involving disadvantaged minority groups and developing nations, can serve two purposes. They can provide data to allow public health professionals to determine and allocate health resources. Cross-cultural studies involving developing countries represent a great opportunity for delineating risk factors for the dementias by providing a much wider diversity of environmental exposures than

* Albert E. Sterne, Professor and Chairman, Department of Psychiatry, Indiana University School of Medicine, 541 Clinical Drive, Room 298, Indianapolis, IN 46202-5111.

R. Mayeux / Y. Christen (Eds.)
Epidemiology of Alzheimer's Disease:
From Gene to Prevention

do studies in industrialized countries, where important risk factors may be missed because of their very pervasiveness. Studies of migrant populations offer an especially good model to explore environmental effects (Osuntokun et al. 1992). The recent findings of a powerful association of genetic risk factors, such as the possession of the ε4 allele of apolipoprotein E and late-onset AD, only serve to enhance the importance of these cross-cultural studies (Corder et al. 1993). Epidemiologists will now be able to combine the techniques of population genetics with environmental risk factor research to explore the interaction between genetics and environment in the etiology of the dementing disorders.

The necessity and advantages of cross-cultural studies have not escaped the attention of policy makers. In 1995 the United States' National Advisory Council on Aging proposed that a major objective for Alzheimer's research should be to "search for selective risk factors through cross-cultural epidemiological studies as a prelude for developing prevention strategies (National Advisory Council on Aging 1995). In 1998, the 14th International Conference on Alzheimer's Disease will be held for the first time in a developing country, India. One of the reasons for this choice was to recognize the universal significance of dementia so that "this understanding and interest will extend to researchers and funding bodies so that findings ... may be generalized to the two thirds of older people who do not live in developed countries" (Prince 1997).

The purpose of this chapter is to discuss studies of dementia and AD which involve bi-ethnic or multi-ethnic comparisons, together with comparative cross-cultural studies involving developing countries or migrant populations. Cross-cultural research is not without controversy, however, particularly regarding the ability of investigators to make valid comparisons of dementia between populations from very different economic and socio-cultural backgrounds. These issues will be discussed in the first section of the chapter.

Methodological Issues

There are many methodological problems in cross-cultural research, particularly when that research involves populations that may be, for the most part, non-literate. Three major issues are construction of a sampling frame, development of culture fair instruments and comparability of diagnoses across sites.

Sampling

In industrialized countries when accurate census data are available, attempts are usually made to derive a representative sample of that population. However, in countries where there is a lack of census data and particularly when rates of the illness studied are likely to be low, a total population survey of a geographically defined area is desirable. As pointed out in the World Health Organization (WHO) protocol for the Research on Aging sampling (WHO 1984), an entire village or well-defined area offers advantages of clear structure homogeneity and decreases the likelihood of missing cases of dementia. The latter technique does, however, have the disadvantage of lack of generalizability. In our Indianapolis-Ibadan Study, both techniques were used. In Indianapolis a representative sample of African Americans was constructed using census data and in Ibadan a total sample of an area of the city of Ibadan (the Idikan wards) was identified (Hall et al. 1996).

Development of Culture Fair Instruments

A major challenge for cross-cultural studies in dementia is the development of culture-fair instruments for assessment. Two basic approaches have been employed. One approach is to develop new instruments based upon the domains of the syndrome of dementia to be measured, viz, memory, language, judgment, etc. The other approach is to start with established instruments and to modify them to that they can be used in the different cultural settings. There is considerable overlap between these two approaches and both have processes in common, including translation, back translation and, most importantly, harmonization. "Harmonization" means that the instrument must be harmonious or consistent with the cultural, linguistic and educational norms of the subject population (Jorm 1990; WHO 1990). There are advantages and disadvantages to both approaches. The establishment of new instruments provides more flexibility in providing for harmonization but the process is more time consuming and the results are not as easily comparable with existing instruments. Modifying existing instruments often means more compromise is necessary in providing harmonization; it is, however, a simpler process and the results are more readily comparable with other studies. Both approaches require the establishment of population norms. The first strategy should lead to a relatively similar distribution of scores in the population to be studied. The second strategy is likely to result in different mean scores in the study populations depending on the individual test characteristics.

Reliable screening instruments based upon cognitive performance are now available which have been used in cross-cultural studies, including the Hindi Mental State Exam (HMSE); Ganguli et al. 1995) and the Cognitive Abilities Screening Instrument (CASI; Teng et al. 1995). In our studies we developed a relatively new screening instrument that included both cognitive testing and informant data about performance in everyday living, the Community Screening Instrument for Dementia (the CSI"D"); Hall et al. 1993, 1996). This instrument has now been used with comparable results (see Table 1) and with good sensitivity and specificity in Caucasian, Cree, African American, Chinese and Yoruba populations. The complicated steps necessary to construct this instrument have been described in previous publications. They included identification of the dementia domains, selection and translation of items from these domains with indigenous investigators, preparation of first drafts for test of acceptability,

Table 1. Mean cognitive scores and informant scores from the CSI"D" in four populations[a]

	N	Cognitive Scores ± SD (Perfect Score = 33)	Informant Scores (Perfect Score = 0)
African American (Indianapolis)	2212	30.4 ± 2.8	2.9 ± 3.4
Yoruba (Ibadan)	2494	28.0 ± 3.8	2.5 ± 2.5
Cree (Manitoba)	179	30.1 ± 2.9	3.1 ± 2.5
English-speaking (Winnipeg)	214	30.26 ± 2.6	2.5 ± 2.8

[a] These scores are not adjusted for education (Hall et al. 1994, 1996). Mean scores from the Jamaican and Chinese populations are now available and will be published shortly.

reviewing and pretesting and pilot testing second drafts and revision of these drafts based upon statistical analysis for use in the major study.

For our clinical evaluation, we decided to use primarily the existing Consortium to Establish a Registry for Alzheimer's Disease (CERAD; Morris et al. 1989) neuropsychological test battery, which again was translated, back translated and harmonized. We now have available normative data for the CERAD subtests for African Americans, Jamaicans and Yoruba (see Table 2, which compares these data with norms from the CERAD studies and from the Monongahela Valley Study; Morris et al. 1989; Unverzagt et al. 1996; Gureje et al. 1995; Unverzagt, personal communication; Gangili et al. 1991).

It must be emphasized that no instrument, even those designed for cross-cultural studies, can be applied to another culture without repeating the process of translation, harmonization and development of normative values for the population to be studied.

Table 2. Group mean values in several CERAD samples[a]

Variable	African American (Unverzagt et al. 1996)	Nigerian (Gureje et al. 1995)	Jamaican (Unverzagt 1998)	Caucasian (Ganguli et al. 1991)	Caucasian (Morris et al. 1989)
n	83	100	72	1350	275
Age	74.6	73.7	79.3	73.1	68.1
Education	10.2	3.6	6.6	12	14.2
Mini-Mental State Exam	27.2[b]	21.3[b]	23.0[b]	27.2[c]	28.9[c]
Animal Fluency	14.4	13.8	9.0	14.2	18.0
Boston Naming Test	12.2	8.2	9.4	14.0	14.6
Constructional Praxis 4	9.0	4.2	6.7	10.5	10.1
Word List Learning (WLL)	14.8	15.2	10.6	18.7	21.1
WLL Delay	4.0	5.7	2.2	7.0	7.2

[a] Group means from much larger numbers of African American and Joruba subjects are now available and will be published shortly.
[b] Mini-Mental State total score based on stating day of the week backwards.
[c] Mini-Mental State total score based on spelling "WORLD" backwards.

Diagnostic Consistency

Diagnostic consistency has been a major issue in all epidemiological research, highlighted recently by the controversy surrounding the apparent large variation in reported prevalence rates of AD (US General Accounting Office 1998). Part of the discrepancies arises from the use of different diagnostic criteria for dementia in epidemiological studies. The effect this would have on reported rates was demonstrated recently by Erkinjuntti et al. (1997), who estimated a 10-fold difference in dementia rates depending upon the use of one of the existing published criteria. Perhaps an even more vexing issue is determining the threshold for severity that has to be reached to justify diagnosis for all criteria of dementia. If this threshold is revised or lowered, the effect would be to include (or not include) subjects in the dementia category that may be considered cognitively impaired (CI) in other studies. In three studies that have reported both CI and dementia, about as many subjects were identified as being CI as being demented (Hendrie 1998). Clearly, in trans-national, cross-cultural studies, attempts to ensure diagnostic consistency become crucial.

To establish diagnostic consistency in our Indianapolis-Ibadan study, the following procedures were developed (Hall et al. 1993, 1996; Hendrie et al. 1995). Prior to the study, faculty from both Indiana and Ibadan participated in WHO-sponsored training programs (Baldereschi et al. 1994). Later the faculty visited each site and participated in clinical evaluation of dementia. The diagnostic process was as follows. Comprehensive neuropsychological, informant, neurological, physical and, where necessary, laboratory data were collected. All subjects were seen by a physician/investigator. A consensus diagnostic conference was then conducted at each site where the health care personnel, including the examining physician, the neuropsychologist, and at least one other senior investigator, reviewed all of the data and arrived at a preliminary diagnosis. Physicians from Indianapolis and Ibadan then made exchange visits to review the clinical data, visit selected subjects and, blind to the preliminary diagnosis, make independent diagnoses. A final consensus conference involving faculty from both sites resolved differences between sites and arrived at the final diagnosis. This type of consensus diagnosis depends obviously on having a group of well-trained physicians at each site.

The Necessity for Longitudinal Studies

Longitudinal studies are essential in cross-cultural research for several reasons. First of all, in developing nations it is likely that mortality rates and survival after the onset of dementia may differ considerably from those in developed nations. The studies of prevalence rates by themselves give only a very limited understanding of true illness rates. For a more thorough understanding, studies of incidence rates are necessary. Secondly, the establishement of baseline measurements of cognition and function make the diagnosis of dementia in subjects who subsequently undergo cognitive decline more valid, i.e., subjects act as their own controls. Thirdly, following patients diagnosed as demented offers an opportunity to test the validity of the original diagnosis by comparing their course to the established course of the disease in other countries. This latter validation process is especially important in epidemiological work in developing nations, where autopsy studies are unlikely.

Multi Ethnic Comparative Studies in Dementia or AD

A summary of 10 studies of dementia that have included bi-ethnic or multiethnic comparisons usually involving comparisons with the dominant indigeneous population is shown in Table 3. Most of these studies took place in the United States but there are a few located in other countries.

Table 3. Multi-ethnic comparative studies in dementia and AD (compared to dominant indigenous population)

Country	Minority population	Type of study	Results	Explanation
United States Schoenberg et al. 1985)	African Americans	Prevalence	↑ African Americans	?
United States (Folstein et al. 1991)	Non-Whites	Prevalence	↑ Non-Whites	?
United States (Gurland et al. 1995)	African Americans and Hispanics	Prevalence	No direct comparisons ↑ African Americans (75–84)	Educational/ sociocultural/ interaction
Unitd States (Tang et al. 1998)	African Americans and Hispanics	Cumulative Risk	↑ African Americans ↑ Hispanics	Genetic/ environmental
United States (Perkins et al. 1997)	African Americans and Hispanics	Prevalence	↑ African American males ↑ Hispanic males	Vascular
United States[a] (Fillenbaum et al. 1998)	African Americans	Prevalence Incidence	No differences	
United States (de la Monte et al. 1989)	African Americans	Autopsy	↑ Vascular dementia ↓ AD	Genetic
United Kingdom (McCracken et al. 1997)	African/ Caribbean Chinese	Prevalence	↑ Non-English-speaking minorities	Language
Israel[a] (Bowirrat et al. 1997)	Arab Israeli	Prevalence	↑ Arab Israeli	– Illiteracy – Genetic – Environmental
Canada (Hendrie et al. 1993)	Cree	Prevalence	↓ Cree for AD	Sociocultural/ environmental

[a] Abstract only available.

Non-United States Studies

The Liverpool Health and Agency (McCracken et al. 1997) study interviewed a randomly sampled cohort of 418 elderly subjects (65 years and over) of varying ethnicity (including Black African, Black Caribbean and Chinese). Prevalence of dementia was estimated using the Geriatric Mental State Exam (GMSE) and the AGECAT and the results were compared with the results from the larger Mental Research Council's (MRC) alpha study. There were no significant differences in prevalence rates between English-speaking ethnic groups and the indigenous populations. Higher levels of dementia were found among non-English-speaking groups but the authors attributed these findings to misinterpretation of items, such as orientation, in these groups.

Bowirrat et al. (1997) reported on a study of 821 elderly Arab subjects, 60 years and over, living in northeast Israel. Evaluations were conducted by an Arab-speaking neurologist and AD was diagnosed using NINCDS-ADRDA criteria. Illiteracy was strongly associated with rates of AD but the prevalence rates within the Arab-Israeli population were still three times higher than among equivalently undereducated people in Israel. The authors conclude that the high rates of AD in Arab-Israelis may be associated with other genetic or environmental factors.

We conducted a two-stage community survey and subsequent clinical examinations of 192 Cree, aged 65 years and over, living on two reserves in Canada and compared the rates of dementia and AD to an age-stratified sample of 241 English-speaking residents of Winnipeg (Hendrie et al. 1993). Prevalence rates for dementia were about the same across populations but the Cree had lower rates of AD. The most striking impression of the investigators in this study was the continuity of intellectual activities of the elderly in the reserves, where the elderly Cree have traditionally occupied the role of the transmitters of cultural learning. A subsequent study of Cherokee Indians (Rosenberg et al. 1995) in the United States raised the interesting possibility that a greater degree of Cherokee ancestry also reduced the risk of AD in that population. These investigators proposed a genetic explanation for these findings, however.

United States Studies

One of the first reports involving bi-ethnic comparisons was from the Copiah County study by Schoenberg et al. (1985). Residents aged 40 years and over of Copiah County in Mississippi (about equal proportion of Black and White) were interviewed and estimates of severe dementia were made by an investigator neurologist. Age-adjusted prevalence rates for chronic progressive dementia (AD?) were somewhat higher (about one and one-half times) in the black population than in the white population. No attempt was made to explain these Black/White differences.

A part of the Epidemiological Catchment Area Program, a three-stage East Baltimore Mental Health Survey, was conducted on a cross-sectional sample of

923 subjects, 65 years and over (Folstein et al. 1991). Two hundred and ten of these subjects were non-White. Non-Whites had about a two-fold higher rate of dementia, both for individuals diagnosed with AD (although the difference was not statistically significant) and for vascular dementia. No explanations were offered for these differences.

Two reports involving multi-ethnic comparisons have been published from the North Manhattan Aging Project. This project identifies cases of AD and related dementias in subjects 65 years and over living in a defined geographical area in North Manhattan, consisting of mixed Latinos, African American and White ethnic groups. Gurland et al. (1995) noted the pervasive effect of low education on increased prevalence rates of dementia across socio-cultural groups. No direct comparisons of prevalence rates were provided by ethnic group but it was noted that high rates of dementia were found in African Americans 75–84 years of age. In a prospective longitudinal study (2.4 years; Tang et al. 1998) of a sample of these North Manhattan subjects (n = 1079; 16.8 % African American, 61.2 % Hispanic and 22 % White), the cumulative risk of AD to age 90 years adjusted for education and sex was four times higher for African Americans and two times higher in Hispanics than in the White population for subjects who did not possess the *APOE* ε4 allele. The investigators suggest that other genes or risk factors may contribute to the increased risk of AD in these minority subjects.

Perkins et al. (1997) conducted a two-stage study of dementia of 564 retired municipal workers in Houston (172 Blacks, 40 Hispanics and 352 Caucasians). Prevalence rates were about two-fold higher among Black and Hispanic men compared to White men, but these differences did not reach statistical significance. The authors suggest that ethnic differences may be due to genetic predisposition or exposure to other putative risk factors such as head injury, drug history or toxics.

In a preliminary report of prevalence and three-year incidence of dementia and AD in a poplation of Blacks and Whites in a five-county, urban/rural area of North Carolina, Fillenbaum et al. (1998) found no differences between ethnic groups in either prevalence or incidence rates for dementia and AD. This study was conducted on a stratified random sample of members of the Duke Established Population for Epidemiological Studies of the Elderly (EPESE; n = 4,136; 55 % Blacks).

There is one report from an autopsy study from 144 consecutive autopsies performed at Johns Hopkins Hospital where a diagnosis of dementia was recorded (78 Whites and 66 Blacks); de la Monte et al. 1989). The frequency of AD was 2.6 times higher in Whites than in Blacks, but multi-infarct dementia and dementia due to alcohol abuse was higher in Blacks. In the same study, in a control group of 100 neurologically normal subjects (50 Blacks and 50 Whites) incidental histological lesions of AD were observed more frequently in Whites than in Blacks. The authors conclude that genetic risk for AD and vascular dementia is different in Blacks and Whites.

Although the majority of studies suggest that minority ethnic groups are at greater risk for developing dementia and AD, considerable discrepancies remain between the reported findings. This is perhaps not surprising when comparing different ethnic groups but it is also found in studies of single ethnic minorities, such as the African Americans. There are several possible reasons for these discrepancies.

The studies vary considerably in methodology, in sampling methods, in reported rates (prevalence, incidence, cumulative risk) as well as in case identification. It might be anticipated that diagnosis of mild dementia, where more reliance is made on neuropsychological tests, may be particularly difficult in ethnic groups because of communication and language problems as well as the availability of normative values (McCracken et al. 1997). However, in the North Manhattan study, differences between the ethnic and White groups persisted even when comparisons were limited to moderate to severe dementia (Tang et al. (1998). One major problem is the sample size in the reported studies. Most have relatively small numbers of subjects in the individual ethnic categories. This fact, together with relatively high refusal rates in minority groups in some studies, makes the reported rates relatively unstable and the corresponding confidence intervals (which are not always given) high. It is likely that there is considerable genetic heterogeneity within ethnic groups for example, in Hispanics or African Americans, based upon their country of origin or from subsequent intermarriage. It is also likely that ethnic groups living in diverse geographic settings are subject of different environmental exposures. Fang et al. (1996) recently demonstrated considerable variation in mortality rates due to cardio-vascular disease within African American populations, depending on their place of birth. It is possible, therefore, that the variation in rates of AD for African Americans in New york and North Carolina may be explained by a combination of genetic and site-specific environmental differences.

Cross National Studies

There have been many studies conducted on the prevalence of dementia and AD throughout the world, although very few have been conducted in non-industrialized countries. These studies have reported widely different prevalence rates but these variations have generally been considered to be due to methodological issues (Graves and Kukull 1993). One persistent finding has been the reported variation in dementia subtypes between Japan, where vascular dementias predominate, and Europe and the United States, where AD predominates (Graves et al. 1993). These differences may be due to lack of agreement about the criteria for vascular dementia between investigators. There have been very productive attempts to combine data from studies from different nations, e.g., the EURODEM project (Brayne 1991), but few international studies have attempted to use identical methodology in multiple sites. One of the pioneering attempts was the United States-United Kingdom Cross-National Geriatric Community Study which found as yet unexplained higher rates of prevalence of dementia in New York than in London (4.9 % in New York, 2.3 % in London; Gurland et al. 1983).

Table 4. Age-standardized prevalence rates of dementia in comparative international studies (Canadian study acting as referrent)[a]

Studies	Criteria	Age composition (Years)	Rates (%)	Predominant subtypes
Ni-Hon-Sea				
Japanese American (Seattle)	DSM-III-R	65+	6.3	AD
Japanese American (Honolulu)	DSM-III-R	Over 70 (men only)	7.6	AD
Japanese (Hiroshima)[b]	DSM-III-R	60+	5.3	AD (in women)
Indianapolis-Ibadan				
African Americans (Indianapolis	ICD-10	65 +	8.24	AD
Yoruba (Ibadan)	ICD-10	65+	2.29	AD
Canadian				
Cross National (English-speaking)	DSM-III-R/ICD-10	65+	8.0	AD

[a] No prevalence rates as yet are available from the Indo-US Study.
[b] Abstract only available.

In this section, three major comparative international studies that use similar methodology and include developing countries and/or migrant populations will be reviewed: the Indo-US Study and two studies of migrant populations, the Ni-Hon-Sea Studies and the Indianapolis-Ibadan project. Table 4 summarizes the prevalence rates for these studies with the results from the large Canadian cross-national study (n = 10,000) added as a reference point (Canadian Study of Health and Aging Working Group 1994).

The Indo-US Cross National Dementia Epidemiology Study

The Indo-US Cross National Dementia Epidemiology Study is a comparative study of the epidemiology of the dementing disorders between an elderly population in a rural district in Northern India and a population of elderly subjects living in the Monongahela Valley in Pennsylvania, USA (MoVIES Project). The investigators have published a number of articles about the methodology and the development of culture fair instruments and also some preliminary findings suggesting that cognitive impairment in India may be related to site-specific, neurological disorders resulting from nutritional deficiencies. No prevalence data on dementia or AD are as yet available from this study (Chandra et al. 1998; Ganguli et al. 1996).

The Ni-Hon-Sea Project

The Ni-Hon-Sea Project consists of a group of independently funded comparative studies of dementia and aging in samples of Japanese populations at three sites: Hiroshima, Japan; Kings County, Washington (The KAME Project); and Oahu, Hawaii. The Hawaiian study is part of the Honolulu Heart Program. These studies, while all independent, have used comparable methodologies, screening and clinical instruments. Prevalence rates for dementia and AD have been published from the Hawaii and Washington sites and preliminary prevalence rates have been reported from Hiroshima (see Table 4; Graves et al. 1996 a, White et al. 1996; Yamada et al. 1997). Both groups of investigations of Japanese-American populations in Seattle and Honolulu have commented on the similarity of their reported rates of dementia and their finding that AD is the predominant dementia subtype and the reported rates from studies of Caucasian populations in North America and Europe, suggesting a strong environmental influence on disease rates. They also commented on the differences between their studies and previously reported studies of dementia in Japan, where vascular dementia predominates. However, in the preliminary results from the Hiroshima study, AD was the predominant dementia subtype for women but in men the rates of AD and vascular dementia (VD) were about equal.

An intriguing preliminary finding from the Seattle-based Japanese-American Study was that preservation of a Japanese lifestyle in subjects was associated with both low levels of cognitive decline and lower rates of AD in that sample (Graves et al. 1996 b).

The Indianapolis-Ibadan Study

Since 1992, research teams from the faculties of Indiana University School of Medicine and the University of Ibadan, Nigeria, have been collaborating on longitudinal comparative studies supported by the National Institute on Aging (NIA) of the prevalence and incidence rates of AD and other dementing illnesses in African Americans residing in Indianapolis and Yoruba living in the Idikan wards in the city of Ibadan. So far, we have reported significant differences in the age-adjusted prevalence rates of dementia (8.24 % in Indianapolis, 2.29 % in Ibadan) and AD (6.24 % in Indianapolis, 1.41 % in Ibadan; Hendrie et al. 1995). These rate differences may possibly be due to differences in dementia survival in our two populations. Whether or not true differences exist will depend upon the analysis of the mortality rates and incidence rates in the two populations, which is now ongoing. There also appears to be a differential association between the possession of the ε4 allele of *APOE* and risk for AD in the two communities. The association in the African Americans was somewhat weaker than that reported for other populations, being evident only in ε4 homozygotes (Sahota et al. 1997). So far, no association between ε4 and dementia and AD has been detected in the Nigerian sample (Osuntokun et al. 1995). These findings raise the possibility of the presence of other factors (environmental or genetic) that reduce the *APOE* ε4 associated risk for AD in populations of African origin. One major difference between sites is diet. This is reflected in mean cholesterol levels, which are much lower in Nigerian subjects than in the African American subjects.

Summary

Cross-cultural, trans-national comparative studies of dementia and AD are in their infancy, but there are already some intriguing findings that may enhance our understanding of the genesis of Alzheimer's disease.

The results from the studies in North Manhattan of African Americans and Hispanics, together with the findings from the Indianapolis-Ibadan studies and the studies of the Cherokees, support the concept that in some ethnic groups – Africans, American Indians, and Hispanics – the constellation of genetic factors responsible for AD may differ from those found in Caucasian populations. This variation in risk association between genetic factors and illness across ethnic groups is not an uncommon phenomenon. It has been reported, for example, that the association between molecular variants of the angiotensinogen gene and hypertension differs in populations of African origin and Caucasian populations (Rotimi et al. 1994). The findings do reinforce the concept that a full understanding of the genetic contribution to AD will require studies in different ethnic groups.

They also highlight the importance of studying other environmental risk factors in the genesis of AD. In the case of the African Americans who are particularly prone to cardiovascular disease, the role that vascular risk factors may play not only in stoke-related dementia but also in AD needs to be explored further. The great differences in diet between the Nigerians and the African Americans and the much lower mean cholesterol levels in the Nigerian subjects suggest that dietary constituents such as fat intake may be risk factors for AD, as has already been proposed in the Rotterdam study (Kalmijn et al. 1997).

Finally, studies also suggest that certain socio-cultural influences, in addition to education, either within cultures or between cultures, may play an important modifying role in the evolution of AD. The preservation of a Japanese lifestyle as an apparently protective factor for cognitive decline, as reported in the *Kame* studies, is one example of this influence. The continuation of the traditional role of the elderly Cree as an explanation for lower rates of AD in that community, as suggested by the Cree community leaders, is another. It is tempting to speculate that other types of cultural interactions and acculturation processes may be particularly stressful and may account for higher rates of illness in these groups, e.g., ethnic minorities in large cities. Socio-cultural hypotheses need to construct a scientifically plausible connection between psychosocial factors and disease pathogenesis, however. Perhaps the recent studies suggesting that aging enhances hypothalamopituitary adrenal axis (HPA) responsivity and that chronic increases in plasma cortisol levels may be implicated in hippocampal damage and cognitive decline provide this link (Lupien et al. 1998).

Dr. Gillum (1996), in an editorial in the *New England Journal of Medicine*, proposed a very sophisticated model of the stages in the epidemiological evolution of patterns of cardiovascular disease among subjects of Sub-Saharan African origin, involving acculturation, urbanization, affluence, saturated fat intake, salt intake and smoking. It is too early in the evolution of the cross-cultural studies of AD to construct similar sophisticated constructs of genetic, environmental and socio-cultural interactions, but there is already considerable promise that these models will be more apparent in the near future.

References

Baldereschi M, Amato MP, Nencini P, Pracucci G, Lippi A, Amaducci L, Gauthier S, Beatty L, Quiroga P, Klassen G, Galea A, Muscat P, Osuntokun B, Ogunniyi A, Portera-Sanchez A, Bermejo F, Hendrie H, Burdine V, Brashear A, Farlow M, Maggi S, Katzman R (1994) Cross-national interrater agreement on the clinical diagnostic criteria for dementia: WHO-PRA Age-Associated Dementia Working Group, WHO Program for Research on Aging, Health of Elderly Program. Neurology 44:239–242

Bowirrat A, Treves TA, Friedland RP, Korczyn AD (1997) Prevalence of dementia of Alzheimer type in an elderly Arab Population: a door-to door survey. In: Abstracts of the Eighth Congress of the International Psychogeriatric Association: Aging in a World of Change, Jerusalem, Israel, August 17–22, p. 74

Brayne C (1991) The EURODEM collaborative re-analysis of case-control studies of Alzheimer's disease: implications for public health. Int J Epidemiol Suppl 2:S175–S177

Canadian Study of Health and Aging Working Group (1994) Canadian Study of Health and Aging: study methods and prevalence of dementia. J Can Med Assoc 150:899–913

Chandra V, DeKosky ST, Pandav R, Johnston J, Belle SH, Ratcliff G, Ganguli M (1998) Neurological factors associated with cognitive impairment in a rural elderly population in India: The Indo-US Cross-National Dementia Epidemiology Study. J Geriat Psych Neurol 11:11–13

Class CA, Unverzagt FW, Gao SJ, Hall KS, Baiyewu O, Hendrie HC (1996) Psychiatric disorders in African-American nursing home residents. Am J Psych 153:677–681

Corder EH, Saunders AM, Strittmatter WJ, Schmechel DE, Gaskell PC, Small GW, Roses AD, Haines JL, Pericak-Vance MA (1993) Gene dose of apolipoprotein E type 4 allele and the risk of Alzheimer's disease in late onset families. Science 261:921–923

de la Monte SM, Hutchins GM, Moore GW (1989) Racial differences in the etiology of dementia and frequency of Alzheimer lesions in the brain. J Nat Med Assoc 81:644–652

Erkinjuntti T, Ostbye T, Steenhuis R, and Hachinski V (1997) The effect of different diagnostic criteria on the prevalence of dementia. New Engl J Med 337:1667–1674

Ernst RL, Hay JW (1996) The US economic and social costs of Alzheimer's disease revisited. Am J Public Health 84:1261–1264

Evans DA, Funkenstein HH, Albert MS, Scherr PA, Cook NR, Chown MJ, Hebert LE, Hennekens CH, Taylor JO (1989) Prevalence of Alzheimer's disease in a community population of older persons. Higher than previously reported. JAMA 262:2551–2556

Fang J, Madhavan S, Alderman MH (1996) The Association between birthplace and mortality from cardiovascular causes among Black and White residents of New York City. New Engl J Med 335:1545–1551

Fillenbaum GG, Heyman A, Huber MS, Woodbury MA, Leiss J, Schmader KE, Bohannon A, Trapp-Moen B (1998) Prevalence and three-year incidence of dementia in older Black and White community residents. Abstract presented at the 1998 American Academy of Neurology Scientific Meeting, April 25–May 2, 1998. Neurology 50(S4):A55

Folstein MF, Bassett SS, Anthony JC, Romanoski AJ, Nestadt GR (1991) Dementia: case ascertainment in a community survey. J Gerontol 46:M132–138

Ganguli M, Ratcliff G, Belle S, Huff FJ, Kancel MJ, Fischer L, Kuller LH (1991) Effects of age, gender, and education on cognitive tests in an elderly rural community sample: norms from the Monongahela Valley Independent Elders Survey (MoVIES). Neuroepidemiology 10:42–52

Ganguli M, Ratcliff G, Chandra V, Sharma S, Gilby J, Pandav R, Belle S, Ryan C, Baker C, Seaberg E, Dekosky S (1995) A Hindi Version of the MMSE: The Development of a cognitive screening instrument for a large illiterate rural elderly population in India. Int J Geriat Psych 10:367–377

Ganguli M, Chandra V, Gilby JE, Ratcliff G, Sharma SD, Pandav R, Seaberg EC, Belle (1996) Cognitive test performance in a community-based nondemented elderly sample in rural India: The Indo-U.S. Cross-National Dementia Epidemiology Study. Int Psychogeriat 8:507–524

Gillum RF (1996) Editorial: The epidemiology of cardiovascular disease in Black Americans. New Engl J Med 335:1597–1599, Nov

Graves AB, Kukull WA (1993) The epidemiology of dementia. In: Morris JC (ed) Handbook of dementing illnesses: New York, Marcel Decker

Graves AB, Larson EB, Edland SD, Bowen JD, McCormick WC, McCurry SM, Rice MM, Wenzlow A, Uomoto JM (1996 a) Prevalence of dementia and its subtypes in the Japanese American population of King County, Washington State: The Kame Project. Am J Epidemiol 144:760–771, Oct

Graves AB, Larson EB, Wenzlow A (1996 b) Protective factors for cognitive decline in a Japanese American community. Abstract presented at The Fifth International Conference on Alzheimer's Disease and Related Disorders. Neurobiol Aging 17(4S):S40

Gureje O, Unverzagt FW, Osuntokun BO, Hendrie HC, Baiyewu O, Ogunniyi A, Hall KS (1995) The CERAD Neuropsychological Test Battery: Norms from a Yoruba-speaking Nigerian sample. West African J Med 14:29–33

Gurland B, Copeland J, Kuriansky J, Kelleher M, Sharpe L, Dean LL (1983) The mind and mood of aging mental health problems of the community elderly in New York and London. New York, The Harworth Press

Gurland B, Wilder D, Cross P, Lantigua R, Teresi J, Barrett V, Stern Y, Mayeux R (1995) Relative rates of dementia by multiple case definitions, over two prevalence periods, in three sociocultural groups. Am J Geriat Psych, 3:6–20

Hall KS, Hendrie HC, Rodgers DD, Prince CS, Pillay N, Blue AW, Brittain HM, Norton JA, Kaufert JN, Nath A, Shelton P, Osuntokun BO, Postl BD (1993) The development of a dementia screening interview in two distinct languages. Int J Meth Psychiat Res 3:62.1–62.14

Hall KS, Ogunniyi AO, Hendrie HC, Osuntokun BO, Hui SL, Musick BS, Rodenberg CA, Unverzagt FW, Gureje O, Baiyewu O (1996) A cross-cultural community based study of dementias: Methods and performance of the survey instrument Indianapolis, U.S.A., and Ibadan, Nigeria. Int J Meth Psych Res 6:129–142

Henderson AS (1988) The risk factors for Alzheimer's disease: a review and a hypothesis. Acta Psych Scand 78:257–275

Hendrie HC (1998) Epidemiology of Dementia and Alzheimer's Disease. Am J Geriat Psych 6:S3–S18

Hendrie HC, Hall KS, Pillay N, Rodgers D, Prince C, Norton J, Brittain H, Nath A, Blue A, Kaufert J, Shelton P, Postl B, Osuntokun B (1993) Alzheimer's disease is rare in Cree. Int Psychogeriat 5:5–14

Hendrie HC, Osuntokun BO, Hall KS, Ogunniyi AO, Hui SL, Unverzagt FW, Gureje O, Rodenberg CA, Baiyewu O, Musick BS, Adeyinka A, Farlow MR, Oluwole SO, Class CA, Komolafe O, Brashear A, Burdine VE (1995) Prevalence of Alzheimer's disease and dementia in two communities: Nigerian Africans and African Americans. Am J Psychiat 152:1485–1492

Jorm AF (1990) Psycho-social correlates. In Jorm, AF: The epidemiology of Alzheimer's disease and related disorders. London Chapman and Hall

Jorm AF, Korten AE, Henderson AS (1987) The prevalence of dementia: a quantitative integration of the literature. Acta Psych Scand 76:465–479

Kalmijn S, Launer LJ, Ott A, Witteman JCM, Hofman A, Breteler MMB (1997) Dietary fat intake and the risk of incident dementia in the Rotterdam study. Ann Neurol 42:776–782

Lupien SJ, de Leon M, de Santi S, Convit A, Tarshish C, Nair NPV, Thakur M, McEwen BS, Hauger RL, Meaney MJ (1998) Cortisol levels during human aging predict hippocampal atrophy and memory deficits. Nature Neurosci 1:69:73

McCracken CFM, Boneham MA, Copeland JRM, Williams KE, Wilson K, Scott A, McKibbin P, Cleave N (1997) Prevalence of dementia and depression among elderly people in Black and ethnic minorities. Brit J Psychiat 171(9):269–273

Morris JC, Heyman A, Mohs RC, Hughes JP, van Belle G, Fillenbaum G, Mellts ED, Clark C, CERAD Investigators (1989) The Consortium to Establish a Registry for Alzheimer's Disease (CERAD). Part I. Clinical and neuropsychological assessment of Alzheimer's disease. Neurology 39:1159–1165

National Advisory Council on Aging (1995) Report to Congress on the scientific opportunities for developing treatments for Alzheimer's disease

Osuntokun GO, Hendrie HC, Ogunniyi AO, Hall KS, Lekwauwa UG, Brittain HM, Norton JA, Oyediran AB, Pillay N, Rodgers DD (1992) Cross-cultural studies in Alzheimer's disease. Ethnicity Disease 2:352–357

Osuntokun BO, Sahota A, Ogunniyi AO, Gureje O, Baiyewu O, Adeyinka A, Oluwole SO, Komolafe O, Hall KS, Unverzagt FW, Hui SL, Yang M, Hendrie HC (1995) Lack of an association between Apolipoprotein E ε4 and Alzheimer's disease in elderly Nigerians. Ann Neurol 38:463–465

Perkins P, Annegers JF, Doody RS, Cooke N, Aday L, Vernon SW (1997) Incidence and prevalence of dementia in a multiethnic cohort of municipal retirees. Neurology 49:44–50

Prince M (1997) The need for research on dementia in developing countries. Trop Med Inter Health 2:993–1000

Rocca WA, Amaducci LA, Schoenberg BS (1986) Epidemiology of clinically diagnosed Alzheimer's disease. Ann Neurol 19:415–424

Rosenberg WR, Richter RW, Risser RP, Taubman K, Prado-Farmer I, Ebalo E, Posey J, Kingfisher D, Dean D, Weiner MF, Svetlik D, Adams P, Honig LS, Cullum CM, Schaefer FV, Schellenberg GD (1995). Genetic factors for the development of Alzheimer's Disease in the Cherokee Indians. Arch Neurol 53:997–1000

Rotimi C, Morrison L, Cooper R, Oyejide C, Effiong E, Ladipo M, Osotemihen B, Ward R (1994) Angiotensinogen gene in human hypertension: lack of an association of the 235T allele among Africen Americans. Hypertension 24:591–594

Sahota A, Yang M, Gao S, Hui SL, Baiyewu O, Gureje O, Oluwole S, Ogunniyi A, Hall KS, Hendrie HC (1997) Apolipoprotein E-associated risk for Alzheimer's disease in the African-American population is genotype dependent. Ann Neurol 42:659–661

Schoenberg BS, Anderson DW, Haerer AF (1985) Severe dementia: prevalence and clinical features in a biracial US population. Arch Neurol 42:740–743

Smith K, Shah A, Wright K, Lewis G (1995) The prevalence and costs of psychiatric disorders and learning disabilities. Brit J Psych I66:9–18

Tang MX, Stern Y, Marder K, Bell K, Gurland B, Lantigua R, Andrews H, Feng L, Tycko B, Mayeux B (1998) The APOE-ε4 allele and the risk of Alzheimer's disease among African Americans, whites, and hispanics. JAMA 278:751–755

Teng EL, Hasegawa K, Homma A, Imai Y, Larson E, Graves A, Sugimoto K, Yamaguchi T, Sasaki H, Chiu D, White LR (1994) The Cognitive Abilities Screening Instrument (CASI): a practical test for cross-cultural epidemiological studies of dementia. Int Psychogeriat 6(1):45–58, Discussion 62

United States General Accounting Office (1998) Alzheimer's disease: estimates of prevalence in the United States. GAO Report #HEHS-98-16

Unverzagt FW, Hall KS, Torke AM, Rediger JD, Mercado N, Gureje O, Osuntokun BO, Hendrie HC (1996). Effects of age, education, and gender on CERAD Neuropsychologal Test performance in an African American sample. Clin Neuropsychol 10:180–190

White L, Petrovitch H, Ross GW, Masaki KH, Abbott RD, Teng EL, Rodriguez BL, Blanchette PL, Havlik RJ, Wergowske G, Chiu D, Foley DJ, Murdaugh C, Curb JD (1996) Prevalence of dementia in older Japanese-American men in Hawaii: The Honolulu-Asia Aging Study. JAMA 276:955–960

World Health Organization (1984) The uses of epidemiology in the study of the elderly. Report of a WHO Scientific Group on the Epidemiology of Aging. WHO Techn Rep Ser 706:9

World Health Organization (1990) Program for Research of Aging, Specific Program: Age-Associated Dementia; Protocol of the Study. Report made by the Steering Committee Meeting for Age-associated Dementias. Florence, January 23–24

Yamada M, Sasaki H, Mimon Y, Kasagi F, Sudor S, Nakamura S, Kodama S (1997) Prevalence of dementia in a fixed Japanese population (The Adult Health Study of the Radiation Effects Research Foundation). Abstract presented at the Fifth International Conference on Alzheimer's Disease. Neurobiol Aging 27(4S):S94

The Implications of Epidemiological Findings for the Prevention of Alzheimer's Disease

C. Brayne[1], C. Dufouil[2], M. A. McGee[3]

Summary

The greatest burden of dementia in the population is in age groups that have shown a marked increase in recent decades, mainly those aged 80 to 84 and mainly women. This rise is due to the increase in the prevalence of dementia with age, coupled with the mortality at older ages. As populations age yet further, there will be increases in those in older age groups, who are at even greater risk of dementia. Any serious attempt at prevention of Alzheimer's disease must be planned with this in mind. Despite difficulties with the definition of dementia and its subtypes, many research studies are contributing important results to this research field. Findings from the population are essential in order to quantify the size of the burden of dementia, how much develops over time and how long people in the demented state are likely to live. Knowledge of the risk factors in the population allows examination of their impact on dementia, and also of the potential to prevent dementia. In the UK population data are available for cross sectional findings from the Medical Research Council study of Cognitive Function and Ageing Study (MRC-CFAS), and for longitudinal findings from the Cambridge City Over 75 Cohort, and from deterministic models of prevalence and survival to calculate incidence. These models can also be used to look at the difference between studies in very contrasting settings, such as the Nigerian and American African studies, in which it can be shown that, despite different prevalence proportions, the same incidence can be created through manipulation of survival of those who are demented compared with those who are not, and by introducing a lag for the development of dementia. The maximum preventability of dementia, given current knowledge of risk, can be assessed by examining how much dementia would disappear if certain risks were eradicated. Studies in progress will provide much of the essential data over the next decade to know what impact preventive efforts might have on the total population, and more specifically on dementia.

[1] Department of Community Medicine, Institute of Public Health, Forvie Site, Robinson Way, Cambridge CB2 2SR, England.

[2] Inserm Unit 360 – Hôpital La Salpétrière, 75651 Paris Cédex 13, France.

[3] MRC Biostatistics Unit, Institute of Public Health, Forvie Site, Robinson Way, Cambridge CB2 2SR, England.

R. Mayeux / Y. Christen (Eds.)
Epidemiology of Alzheimer's Disease:
From Gene to Prevention

Introduction

Classical epidemiology provides evidence about the association of putative risk factors with a disease of interest. This approach has worked well with a variety of chronic diseases, usually those that have clearly defined exposures such as smoking, and with clearly defined diseases, such as lung cancer. With Alzheimer's disease, both measurement of the risks and a clear definition of the disease itself present challenges to researchers. For many years the only risk research in Alzheimer's disease was based on comparing cases of Alzheimer's disease with non-demented controls, and these studies failed to identify consistent risks apart from age and family history. Then, paralleling a flowering of research into pathological mechanisms, there has been a regeneration of interest in the wider risks for dementia, cognitive decline and the recognition that longitudinal population-based studies complement the intensive concentration on molecular biological mechanisms of Alzheimer's disease. Even so, studies have not yet provided definitive evidence of which, if any, preventive strategies will reduce the population burden of dementia of Alzheimer's disease in the future.

This presentation concentrates on UK data on the quantification of the burden now and in the near future, the age relationship of dementia, deterministic models and the amount of prevention possible.

Defining the Disorder

Whilst a case of Alzheimer's disease at a young age is very clearly different from the patient's peer group, the difference becomes less marked as age increases, and the probability of dementia becomes much higher. At younger ages the nature of the dementia process will be clearer, in that vascular aetiology is more dramatic and the behavioural and psychotic manifestations of frontal or Lewy body dementia are more obvious, separating these conditions out from the more classical features of Alzheimer's disease. At older ages the distinguishing features of each type of dementia become blurred by the ageing process itself and the frequency of co-morbidity. The difficulty was highlighted in a recent study comparing different criteria, in which very different proportions of a population were declared demented according to widely used different criteria (Erkinjuntti et al. 1997). Thus definitions of dementia remain rather vague, with a reliance on evidence of change beyond socioculturally accepted norms for the age group under study. Many prospective studies have shown consistently that the best early predictors of subsequent cognitive decline and dementia are cognitive measures, particularly verbal memory (Brayne et al. 1997 a).

Quantifying Dementia in the Population

Differentiating Alzheimer's disease from other dementias, and dementia from general ageing, is still not possible without considerable misclassification. Attempts to quantify the size of the problem have been useful to emphasise that this is a syndrome that is costly to society and deserving of a concentration of research effort. Quantification of the size of the problem has been tackled in many settings. From a service provision perspective, measures of established dementia are essential for planning. This fact has reinforced the emphasis on definitions of caseness and identification of discrete types of dementia diagnosis. In the United Kingdom, the Multicentre Study of Cognitive Function and Ageing confirms the known pattern with age in the prevalence of dementia and cognitive impairment (MRC-CFAS 1998), providing similar proportions in the oldest age groups to the previous combined estimates from Europe (Hofman et al. 1994). By using prevalence estimates and known survival patterns in those who are demented compared to those who are not in order to calculate incidence, we showed that the incidence of dementia, mainly Alzheimer's disease in the oldest age groups (Brayne et al. 1995 a), must continue to rise inexorably (McGee and Brayne 1998). Projecting forward in time shows that, assuming no prevention alters the patterns of disease, a considerable rise in the numbers of demented people can be expected due to the differential rise in those aged over 85 (Melzer et al. 1997).

Aetiological studies have been conducted, in the main, on the younger old populations and have limited relevance to the great burden of dementia. Relatively few longitudinal studies have concentrated on the oldest age groups. Volunteer studies at such ages tend to be biased towards the healthy old, and loss to longitudinal population studies can cause considerable bias. Cambridge City has a longitudinal study of the 75 and over age group which has provided insight into the extent of cognitive decline in this age group (Brayne et al. 1995 b), the incidence of dementia (Paykel et al. 1994) and dementia subtypes (Brayne et al. 1995 a) and the neuropathology accompanying decline (Gertz et al. 1998). The neuropathological arm of the study shows a mixture of pathologies, including macrovascular, microvascular lesions, tangles and plaques, and general atrophy in these very old age groups (Brayne et al. 1997 b) which suggest that concentration on the single entity Alzheimer's disease is misguided for the oldest age groups. Strategies examining changes along the dimensional measures that constitute the domain of dementia diagnosis are more appropriate given the difficulty of accurate identification of single underlying processes.

Types of prevention

Prevention can be divided into primary, secondary and tertiary activities. Primary prevention is the avoidance of causative agents of disease; secondary is detecting the disease at an early enough stage to prevent the clinical manifestation of the disease; and tertiary prevention is preventing the consequences of the disease. In each case, the natural history, not only risks and treatments but also matching effective interventions must be known and understood.

Tertiary and Secondary

In dementia most research effort (commercial sector and public sectors) is directed towards finding therapeutic interventions that might be effective in tertiary prevention of established disease. In addition many calls have been made for screening of the older population for dementia in order to detect the small number of dementias that may be caused by reversible disorders such as hypothyroidism, or to set in place management plans at a relatively early stage in the disease progression. But tertiary prevention can only have a limited effect on population burdens of dementia, and secondary prevention similarly so – even if effective methods of screening and treatment were found – since both strategies are based on altering the natural history in the established disease process.

Primary Prevention

Theoretically primary prevention of dementia could be approached from four angles, none of which are mutually exclusive. These are genetic, early, mid and later life approaches.

Several mutations have been established that are associated with Alzheimer's disease in families where several members develop early-onset disease. As high risk individuals with known mutations these families and individuals require services and counselling more akin to the services available for Huntington's chorea. Some laboratories are providing a research service for screening for mutations in, for example, the presenilins to the general community. The only genetic finding that is so far relevant to the older population is the finding that the allelic variations of the apolipoprotein E allele (2, 3 and 4) are associated with varying risk of dementias (Alzheimer's disease has been examined mainly, but the risk appears to be non-specific in that it is associated with other dementias, too). Whether this risk is mediated through a microvascular effect or through the classical Alzheimer's pathology is not yet clear, which may have implications for future action for individuals who are considered to be at greater risk. Much more data are required from longitudinal population studies linked to neuropathological studies before any valid assessment of risk conferred by such genetic findings can be made. In addition, the predictive value from early life of possessing an E4 allele must be much better understood

One theory on the expression of dementia in life is that there is a reserve capacity in the brain, and that the greater this capacity is the later the dementia will be expressed, given a certain level of brain pathology. There are some data to back this theory up, but it is mainly based on clinical studies. Epidemiological studies (mainly case control studies) provide some confirmation that brain size might protect from dementia. Studies in later life examining the impact of educational level show that cognitive impairment, and possibly dementia, are associated with lower levels of attainment. Our own data suggest cognitive decline is not accelerated by low education but that the starting point is lower.

Whether increasing the brain reserve through adequate intrauterine and early life nutrition and maximising it through high levels of education would prevent dementia in the population is not known. The only comparative studies with the same methodologies which show dramatic differences in the prevalence of dementia are those that have measured African American populations and Nigerians. But the findings are converse to the expected, in that the more educated group in America has a higher prevalence of dementia than the Nigerians. In addition there are many other potential confounders, such as survival differences and likelihood of vascular disease, which differ in these populations. Even so, the pattern of rise with age in the Africans is the same as in African Americans, and using a deterministic model, it can be shown that, by introducing a short time lag for the onset of dementia and increasing the likelihood of dying in those who are demented, the Nigerian and African American incidence rates can be made the same (McGee and Brayne 1998).

There is no definitive evidence that maintaining an active intellectual life prevents dementia. It may be desirable for other reasons, such as quality of life, and it may influence the nature and stage of presentation for care or treatment. Reducing vascular risk through the variety of methods promoted widely, such as physical activity, cessation of smoking, moderate but not excessive alcohol intake and balanced nutrition with adequate micronutrient intake, is likely to reduce vascular disease in the brain as well as in the rest of the body (partly through the reduction of late onset Type II diabetes.). These measures are also likely to increase survival, particularly in men, with the consequence that a greater proportion of the old will survive into the at-risk age groups for dementia.

Active treatments that may influence later expression of dementia and may be relevant in middle life are hormone replacement therapy and anti-inflammatory medication intake. Longitudinal studies indicate that some protection is conferred in individuals taking such medication. This finding has yet to be confirmed in randomised controlled trials, which will be reporting over the next few years and are discussed in other chapters.

Adverse exposure to toxins such as aluminium has been shown to cause some neurotoxicity and has been associated with Alzheimer's disease, but not definitively. A general awareness of this association has led to a reduction in the use by some of aluminium cooking utensils, but aluminium is still added to water supplies, is used in antiperspirants and as a food additive and exposure is still widespread. Other toxins such as lead and mercury have been mentioned in the literature but there is no compelling evidence to suggest they are implicated in dementia in the population.

The possibilities for prevention from middle life continue into later life. Preventive strategies for all these areas continue to be effective in later life. Primary prevention of stroke will prevent vascular dementia so that effective treatment of

Table 1. Impact of Prevention. Selected risks from MRC-CFAS (self-reported)

	% of Population reporting risk factor			
	65–74 years		75+ years	
	Men	Women	Men	Women
Head injury	18	8	8	7
HBP	32	37	25	34
Angina	16	10	16	14
Heart attack	15	6	14	9
Stroke	6	4	11	8
Diabetes	6	5	8	6

hypertension is important, bearing in mind that hypotensive episodes are likely to be damaging in their own right. There is no evidence to suggest that antihypertensive treatment causes cognitive decline. The prevention of mortality after first stroke or stroke after transient ischaemic attacks will lead to an increase in the vulnerability to cognitive deficit in the surviving population.

MRC-CFAS data on self-reported vascular risks are shown in Table 1; Parker et al. 1998). These range in importance, and any preventive potential will depend on the size of the risk associated with dementia and the proportion of the population exposed to or suffering from the risk at the appropriate age. Assuming an instant preventive effect and assuming uniformity of effect in all age groups, the proportion of cases prevented can be calculated and varies considerably (Table 2). However, these calculations are very simplistic and preventive effort is likely to lead to other population changes, such as increase in survival.

Considering this evidence on prevention in the context of the population and neuropathological observational data, the following conclusions can be drawn. Secondary and tertiary prevention attempt to halt a process that is already ongoing. At advanced ages other, parallel processes, are also proceeding which may make any such preventive action less effective. These strategies are likely to reduce the societal burden only marginally. Secondary prevention also presupposes accurate differentiation of specific processes at an early stage of the disease. Primary prevention is the most likely strategy to alter age-specific patterns

Table 2. Potential reduction in dementia through preventive measures %

	% exposure				
Relative Risk	5	10	15	20	25
0.5	3	5	7	10	15
0.75	1	2	4	5	6
1.25	1	2	4	5	6
1.50	2	5	7	9	11
2.0	5	9	13	17	20
4.0	13	23	31	37	43

of dementia. The cognitive decline linked to vascular disease is likely to be the most amenable to intervention. Prevention can be implemented at all life stages. Encouraging results from selected longitudinal studies suggest some preventive potential from some micronutrients, oestrogen (for women) and anti-inflammatory medication, but whether such findings will be borne out in trials in the appropriate age groups over relevant time periods has yet to be shown. The next few years will see many research studies come to fruition, providing many results answering the uncertainties discussed here.

References

Brayne C, Gill C, Huppert FA, Barkley C, Gehlaar E, Girling DM, O'Connor D, Paykel ES (1995 a) Incidence of clinically diagnosed subtypes of dementia in an elderly population. Cambridge Project for Later Life. Brit J Psych 167:255–262.

Brayne C, Gill C, Paykel ES, Huppert FA, O'Connor D (1995 b) Cognitive decline in an elderly populations – a two wave study of change. Psychol Med 25:673–683

Brayne C, Huppert FA, Xuereb JH, Gertz HJ, Chi LY, McGee MA, Paykel ES, Harrington C, Mukaetova-Ladinska E, O'Sullivan A, Dening T, Freer C, Wiscik CM (1997 a) An epidemiological study of the dementias in Cambridge: from clinical progression to neuropathology. In: Iqbal K, Winblad B, Nishiruma T, Takeda M, Wisniewski HM (eds) Alzheimer's disease: biology, diagnosis and therapeutics. John Wiley & Sons, Chichester, pp 11–20

Brayne C, Best N, Muir M, Richards SJ, Gill C (1997 b) Five-year incidence and prediction of dementia and cognitive decline in a population sample of women aged 70–79 at baseline. Int J Geriat Psych 12:1107–1118

Erkinjuntti T, Ostbye T, Steenhuis R, Hachinski V (1997) The effect of different diagnostic criteria on the prevalence of dementia. New Engl J Med 337:1667–1674

Gertz HJ, Xueraeb JH, Huppert FA, Brayne C, McGee MA, Paykel ES, Harrington C, Mukaetova-Ladinska E, Arendt T, Wiscik CM (1998) Examination of the validity of the hierarchical model of neuropathological staging in normal ageing and Alzheimer's disease. Acta Neuropathol 95:154–158

Hofman A, Rocca W, Brayne C, Breteler C, Clarke M, Cooper B, Copeland JRM, Dartigues JF, da Silva Droux A, Hagnell O, Heeren TJ, Engedal K, Jonker C, Lindesay J, Lobo A, Mann AH, Mölsa PK, Morgan K, O'Connor DW, Sulkava R, Kay DWK, Amaducci L (1991) The prevalence of dementia in Europe: a collaborative study of 1980–1990 findings. Int J Epidemiol 20:736–748

McGee MA, Brayne C (1998) The impact on prevalence of dementia in the oldest age groups of differential mortality patterns: a deterministic approach. Int J Epidemiol 27:87–90

Melzer D (1997) New drug treatment for Alzheimer's disease: lessons from healthcare policy. Brit Med J 316:762–764

MRC-CFAS (1998) Cognitive function and dementia in six areas of England and Wales: the distribution of MMSE and prevalence of GMS organicity level in the MRC CFA Study. Psychol Med 28:319–335

Parker CJ, Morgan K, Dewey ME and the analysis group of the MRC CFA study (1997) Physical illness and disability among elderly people in England and Wales: the Medical Research Council cognitive function and ageing study. J Epidemiol Community Health 51:494–501

Paykel ES, Brayne C, Huppert FA, Gill C, Barkley C, Gehlaar E, Beardsall L, Girling DM, Pollitt P, O'Connor D (1994) Incidence of dementia in a population older than 75 years in the United Kingdom. Arch Gen Psych 51:325–332

The Primary Prevention of Alzheimer's Disease: Should We Develop Large-Scale Trials?

*D. A. Evans**

Summary

Because the occurrence of Alzheimer's disease is strongly related to age, and the oldest population age groups of all developed countries are continuing to increase in size, the impact of the disease on public health will continue to grow. Improved treatment for persons who have the disease and support for their families are necessary, but by themselves are insufficient to confront a problem of this magnitude; a strategy for primary prevention of the disease is required as well. Prevention strategies must consider the possibility that Alzheimer's disease does not have any single cause but, like many common chronic diseases, is affected by a complex array of risk factors, and that the effects of each of these factors on risk of disease may be small to moderate in magnitude. Changes in risk of this magnitude would have great potential for prevention, but will likely be beyond the ability of even state-of-the-art observational studies to resolve. It is highly likely that randomized controlled trials of adequate size and design will be necessary to definitively assess whether such factors as use of estrogens, antioxidant agents and non-steroidal anti-inflammatory agents protect against Alzheimer's disease, and strong consideration should be given to conducting large-scale trials in the near future. Otherwise, we will likely face continuing uncertainty as to the role of these and other factors in the prevention of the disease, with conflicting results from even the best designed observational studies.

The case of prevention of Alzheimer's disease

The case for prevention as a central strategy against Alzheimer's disease rests on two issues: the severity of the public health problem posed by the disease and the benefits of prevention over cure in confronting a public health problem of this magnitude.

* Rush University and Rush Institute for Health Aging, 1645 W. Jackson Blvd., Chicago, Illinois, USA.

R. Mayeux / Y. Christen (Eds.)
Epidemiology of Alzheimer's Disease:
From Gene to Prevention

The magnitude of the public health problem posed by Alzheimer's disease

Estimates of the incidence or prevalence of Alzheimer's disease in the general population have varied widely, with much of the variation due to difference in study methods. Alzheimer's disease typically does not occur as a sudden event. Instead it usually arises gradually, by minute degrees. Thus, the precise dividing point between normality and Alzheimer's disease is not a matter of secure agreement, and different investigators, each using intelligence and good judgment, will place this dividing point at different locations along the continuum between normality and disease. This fact produces substantial variation in disease incidence and prevalence estimates across studies, especially in the general population, in whom it is commonly difficult to separate, with certainty, mild disease from normality is common. Further, the clinical distinction between Alzheimer's disease and vascular dementia can be difficult and is made differently across studies. Studies that assign a higher proportion of persons with dementia to a diagnosis of Alzheimer's disease will often have a correpondingly lower proportion with vascular dementia. Other factors also contribute to variation in estimates of the occurrence of Alzheimer's disease. The disease is typically not well detected in the usual delivery of health care, with only a fraction of the disease in the general population diagnosed and recorded in the health care system. Brief tests of cognitive function are frequently used as screening tests for Alzheimer's disease in general population studies, with detailed clinical evaluation for the disease restricted to persons who fail the brief screening test, while persons who pass the test are assumed to be free from Alzheimer's disease. The sensitivity of these brief cognitive tests as screening tests is highly imperfect, however, and a number of persons with the disease will remain in the group of persons who pass the test and are excluded from evaluation for disease. The resulting underestimate of incidence or prevalence of disease can be substantial, especially if the group excluded from evaluation is large. Thus, studies that include mild as well as severe disease, use uniform standard evaluation to detect disease, rely on evaluation of the entire population or of a random sample of all population groups and diagnose vascular dementia less readily will produce higher estimates of incidence and prevalence of Alzheimer's disease. Studies that are restricted to severe disease, rely on health-care systems to detect disease directly or indirectly (through use informant report), exclude persons who pass brief screening tests and diagnose vascular dementia more readily will typically produce lower estimates of prevalence or incidence of Alzheimer's disease.

While these variations in methods affect estimates of the absolute numbers of persons in the general population with Alzheimer's disease, the rationale underlying greatly increased efforts toward prevention is much more strongly dependent on the future growth in the number of persons with Alzheimer's disease. This anticipated growth is strongly dependent on the aging of the populations in developed countries, not on estimates of the absolute number of persons affected. As much as they differ in terms of estimating the absolute number of persons with the disease, there is strong agreement about the very strong associ-

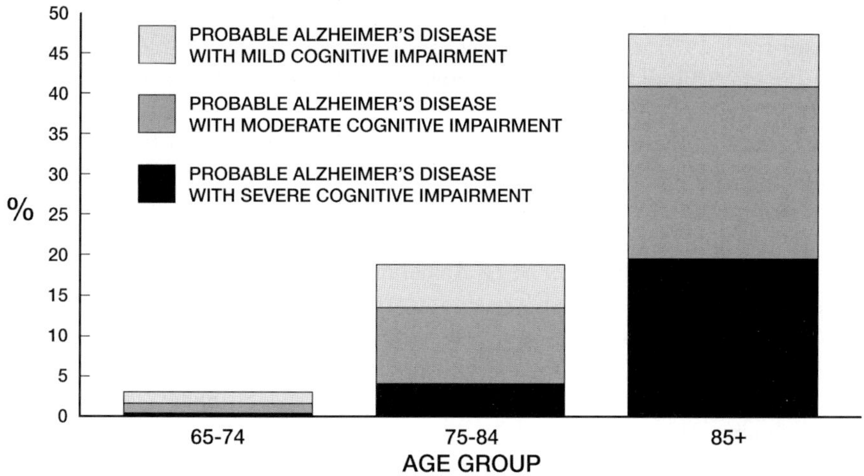

Fig. 1. Prevalence of Alzheimer's disease among community residents 65 and older by age and severity of cognitive impairment. Data from East Boston studies

ation between increasing age and the occurrence of Alzheimer's disease. Further evidence that the strength of the association between Alzheimer's disease and age does not appear to depend on the dividing point used to separate disease and normality may be seen in Figure 1. This graph shows the association between prevalence of Alzheimer's disease and age found in the East Boston Studies, which have provided one of the higher estimates of disease prevalence. The total height of each bar represents the prevalence of disease in each age group, if all levels of disease severity are included. Each bar is also subdivided according to three levels of severity of cognitive impairment: mild, moderate and severe. The high prevalence in the oldest age group, those 85 years of age and older, is not due to a relative excess of mild cases that might be difficult to separate from normality. Instead, the marked increase in prevalence with age is seen for each criterion of disease severity.

The implications of this age distribution for the future public health impact of Alzheimer's disease arise from the rapid aging of the populations of almost all developed countries. Sweden, France, Japan and the United States will experience striking increases in the percents and absolute numbers of persons 80 years of age and older in their populations. In 1970, Sweden and France had the greatest proportions of residents over the age of 80 years, 2.3 %, and this proportion will grow for both countries, somewhat more for Sweden. Growth of the oldest population age groups is expected to be especially striking for Japan; the percent of persons over the age of 80 years was 0.9 % in 1970, but is expected to increase to over 9 % by 2025. The oldest age groups in the population in the United States will experience more moderate growth; the proportion over the age of 80 years is expected to increase from 1.8 % in 1970 to 4.3 % in 2025. The common feature of these patterns is the strong increase in the size of the oldest population groups, both as a percent of the total population and in absolute size. The expected increases from 1970 to 2025 will range from approximately 10-fold in Japan to 2.4-fold in the United States, but the effects on the expected increases in prevalence in Alzheimer's disease will be large for each country. Figures 2 and 3 more closely examine the implications for the change in prevalence of Alzheimer's disease for the United States population (Evans et al. 1990). This may be considered a somewhat moderate situation because, of the four countries shown, the United States population over 80 years of age will experience the least increase. Figure 2 uses estimates of the prevalence of Alzheimer's disease from the East Boston studies projected to the United States population after adjustment for differences in the distribution of age, sex and education, and then projects the number of persons in the United States population with Alzheimer's disease to the year 2050 using three different United States Bureau of the Census estimates, the low, middle and high series. These estimates of population growth vary according to assumptions regarding death, migration and fertility. The growth in the number of persons with Alzheimer's disease is striking for each of the three estimates. Figure 3 repeats the projection of the number of persons with Alzheimer's disease using the middle series estimate and separates the contributions to the overall increase from each of three age groups. The number of persons with Alzheimer's disease in the 65- to 74-year-old group will remain fairly constant. The number of persons with the disease in the 75- to 84-year-old group will increase

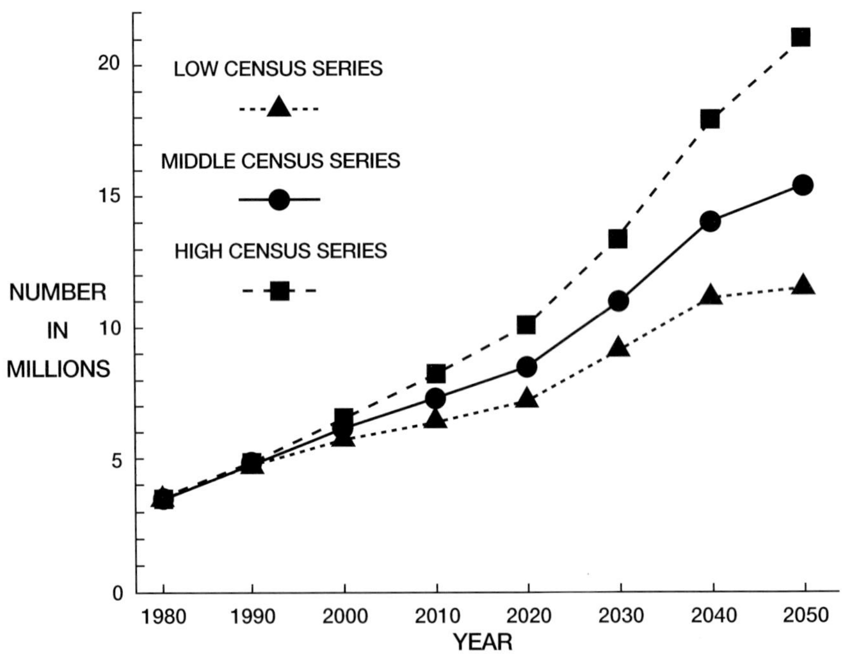

Fig. 2. Change in prevalence of Alzheimer's disease in the United States using three different United States Bureau of Census estimates, the low, the middle and high series

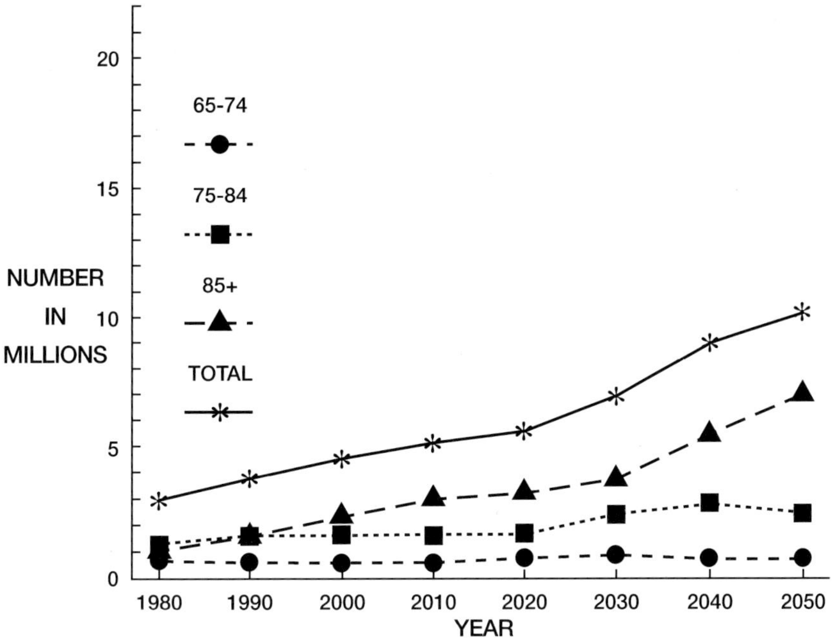

Fig. 3. Projection of the number of persons with Alzheimer's disease using the middle series estimates

moderately, but the overall increase in the number of persons with Alzheimer's disease is clearly being driven by the large increase in the number of persons from the group that are over the age of 85 years.

Prevention and Treatment

Persons with Alzheimer's disease clearly deserve the best of treatment, and strong efforts are warranted to develop drugs that are more effective in limiting or reversing the effects of the disease on cognition. Similarly strong efforts are needed to understand and ameliorate the devastating effects of the disease on the lives of family members of affected persons. Efforts toward treatment of persons with the disease and support of their families should continue and increase but, no matter how strong or successful they are, such efforts will likely not be sufficient to confront a public health problem of the magnitude of Alzheimer's disease. The case for emphasizing prevention as preferable to treatment can be viewed from both economic and humanitarian perspectives. From an economic point of view, the costs of Alzheimer's disease to individuals and society have been estimated only inexactly and with substantial variation, but are very large by any criterion. It seems likely that effective measures to prevent Alzheimer's disease would result in great monetary savings, especially in reduction of use of long-term care. Economic arguments for prevention of other disease have not always been fully borne out, however. Especially if the effect of a preventive measure is to delay the onset of the disease rather than to fully prevent the condition, it can be argued that prevention will result in increased rather than decreased health care costs. Alzheimer's disease, on average, occurs at ages when death due to other cases is frequent and, at least with current life expectancies, delay of disease onset may have the same effects as true prevention. It must be acknowledged, however, that at our current knowledge of the effects of potential preventive measures, economic arguments for the prevention of Alzheimer's disease must be approached with at least some caution. Overall, the strongest argument for prevention is a humanistic one. It was summarized well by Geoffrey Rose: "It is better to be healthy than ill or dead. That is the beginning and the end of the only real argument for preventive medicine. It is sufficient." (Rose 1992).

Identifying Preventive Measures

Is Alzheimer's Disease of Multi-factorial Etiology?

Design of efforts to prevent Alzheimer's disease must take into account the likelihood that, instead of being due to a single cause, the condition, like many other common chronic diseases, is of multi-factorial etiology. Many investigators would agree with MacMahon and Trichopoulos: "If a disease appears to have a single principal cause, it is for one of two reasons: Either we *know* of only one cause, or we have *defined* the disease in terms of a single cause ..." (MacMahon and Trichopoulos 1996). Direct experience with Alzheimer's disease also may be seen as arguing for a complex multi-factorial origin of the disease. Recent research suggests that many factors, in addition to age, may increase or decrease risk of the disease, including level of education or of other markers of socioeconomic status, exposures or experiences during childhood or early adulthood, blood pressure and other vascular factors, use of estrogens, use of non-steroidal anti-inflammatory agents and use of anti-oxidants. While some of the observed associations may be disproved by future studies, the range of risk factors is consistent with experience with other common conditions. The effects of any one of these factors on overall risk of disease may be small, but because of the large public health problem posed by Alzheimer's disease, the preventive implications of validly identifying a factor with even a modest effect on disease risk may be substantial if exposure to the factor can be modified.

Observational Studies

The likelihood of a multi-factorial "web of causation" (MacMahon and Trichopoulos 1996) for Alzheimer's disease places large demands on studies, in that they must be able to validly identify small to moderate changes in risk. Studies to identify risk factors with potential for intervention may be somewhat arbitrarily divided into three general classes: case-control studies of Alzheimer's disease, typically with cases identified through receipt of health care at a clinic or other medical facility; longitudinal studies of Alzheimer's disease, often conducted as large-scale population studies of disease incidence; and randomized clinical trials with occurrence of Alzheimer's disease as the primary outcome, as distinguished from randomized trials of treatments for persons who already have Alzheimer's disease. In general case-control studies have had difficulty in validly identifying risk factors for Alzheimer's disease. Sources of difficulty have included accurate collection of information about risk factors retrospectively from informants after the onset of disease and, perhaps even more importantly, ability to identify truly comparable control individuals for comparison to the persons with Alzheimer's disease identified through clinical sources. The latter issue is especially difficult because the persons identified as having Alzheimer's disease clinically represent a small, and very likely non-random, fraction of all persons with the disease. On average, persons receiving health care for a disease may differ systematically from those with unrecognized disease according to many factors, including age, socioeconomic status, social networks, and severity and clinical features of the disease, and some of these factors affecting recognition of the disease may also affect risk of the disease. Longitudinal observational studies of incident disease, especially large-scale studies in defined populations, have been important in identifying risk factors for many common chronic conditions and have contributed substantially to our knowledge of Alzheimer's disease. These studies offer two general advantages over case-control studies: ability to collect risk factor information for all members of a cohort prior to the onset of overt disease, and potential to ascertain the presence or absence of the disease uniformly for the cohort.

Despite these advantages, longitudinal population-based studies of incident Alzheimer's disease also must confront limitations. Many of the risk factors of interest in the prevention of Alzheimer's disease are related to one another. For example, use of estrogens among older women is inversely related to age and positively related to education and other markers of socioeconomic status. To accurately assess the relation of use of this hormone to disease incidence, it is necessary to separate its potential effects from any confounding effects of age and education. Although this can be done by statistical adjustment, it is difficult to be sure that a study has measured each of the factors precisely enough to permit completely adequate adjustment. As the magnitude of the potential risk associated with a factor becomes smaller, it becomes more difficult to definitively separate any true effect from the possibility of residual confounding by other variables associated with the disease, both the variables about which one knows, and the possibility of confounding by unknown and unmeasured confounding variables. The magnitude of many of the risks that may be important to the prevention of Alzheimer's disease will likely be beyond the ability of even state-of-the-art observational studies to resolve definitively.

Developing Strategies for the Primary Prevention of Alzheimer's Disease: The Role of Randomized Trials

The issue of whether to develop and implement a strategy for the primary prevention of Alzheimer's disease at this time deserves careful consideration. Randomized trials are not the only component of a strategy for prevention; successful primary prevention efforts will require continued emphasis on basic laboratory work to provide the knowledge of pathogenesis on which preventive measures can be based, and even greater emphasis on observational epidemiological studies, especially large-scale longitudinal, population-based studies. Randomized trials are, however, an essential component of an effective primary prevention strategy. One of the key advantages of randomized trials over observational studies is that randomization in a trial of adequate size and design offers potentially complete control of confounding. Adequate randomization assures that, on average, confounding factors will be equally distributed in the intervention and non-intervention groups, and that this will apply not only to known confounding factors but to any confounding factors that are present but unsuspected at the time the trial is conducted. For effects of moderate to small size that have potential public health importance, "the results of a randomized trial will yield the most direct epidemiologic evidence on which to base a judgment of whether an observed association is one of cause and effect." (Hennekens and Buring 1987).

Points may be raised for and against trials of primary prevention of Alzheimer's disease at this time. Perhaps the most compelling argument for them flows from the combination of the public health problem posed by the disease, which is large and continuing to grow, and the possibility that further large-scale observation studies of rigorous design will provide only equivocal and variable evidence regarding some factors of potential importance, because the effects of these factors are sufficiently small that they are difficult to separate from residual confounding. Points arguing against primary prevention trials at this time include their complexity, costs and the possibility that they may draw resources away from other research projects in the field. A crucial issue is whether we have preventive measures with sufficient support from laboratory, clinical and observational epidemiologic studies to warrant testing in randomized trials. As important but often conflicting findings emerge suggesting that some agents may have potential to partially prevent or delay onset of the disease, the questions facing the field are not whether trials of primary prevention should be conducted but are questions of timing and emphasis. For which agents do findings of potential efficacy and low risk warrant randomized trials of primary prevention now or in the near future? The large and growing public health and economic impacts of Alzheimer's disease constitute a firm rational basis for continued expansion of research funding, but can this funding be expanded sufficiently rapidly in the near future to cover the costs of large scale trial without impairing funding in other areas?

The most likely candidates for large-scale trials of primary prevention of Alzheimer's disease may be estrogens, non-steroidal anti-inflammatory agents and anti-oxidant vitamin supplements, especially vitamin E. For each of these three interventions, laboratory studies are available that suggest a plausible mechanism of action that could partially prevent or delay the onset of Alzheimer's disease. The base of observational studies suggesting that persons who use the agent are at lower risk of Alzheimer's disease than are persons who do not is probably strongest for use of estrogens, intermediate for non-steroidal anti-inflammatory drugs and least well developed for anti-oxidant nutrients. On the other hand, a treatment trial indicates that one anti-oxidant nutrient, vitamin E, slows progression of some aspects of Alzheimer's disease, and anti-oxidants appear to have lower toxicity than either estrogens or non-steroidal anti-inflammatory agents. The first large-scale trials of estrogen in primary prevention of Alzheimer's disease have begun, and trials of other agents, such as non-steroidal anti-inflammatory agents, are at the stage of being planned or proposed.

A central feature of the rationale for randomized trials outlined previously is that Alzheimer's disease is likely to be of multi-factorial etiology and that most risk factors and preventive measures are likely to modify risk of disease only slightly or moderately. It follows that, at best, the results of any single primary prevention trial will lead to incomplete prevention or delay in onset of the disease. Even small or moderate reductions in disease occurrence would be of substantial public health importance, however, and the vision for an overall prevention strategy would be to achieve a major reduction in the occurrence of the disease in incremental steps, as individual risk factors and preventive measures are identified, the same strategy that has been effective in lowering risk of other common chronic diseases such as coronary heart disease. Thus, beginning to conduct large-scale trials of primary prevention of Alzheimer's disease is probably best seen not as a leap that will soon lead to dramatic reductions in occurrence of the disease but as starting down a path that will ultimately reach this goal. This path is also likely to pass through some difficult regions. Our knowl edge of the pathogenesis of Alzheimer's disease remains uncertain, but disease prevention does not always require a full understanding of the etiology of the disease. For example, sterilization of needles was identified as an important means of reducing risk of hepatitis long before the etiologic agents were described clearly. Because it is not possible to identify risk factors and preventive measures with certainty from the results of observational studies, it is very likely that some expensive and time-consuming primary prevention trials will produce only null results, while others are highly successful. The motivation to carry out randomized prevention trials Alzheimer's disease should probably arise not from any anticipation of rapid sweeping success but from fear of the consequences of waiting too long to use this means of confronting a disease that poses such a large threat to public health.

References

Evans DA, Scherr PA, Cook NR, Albert MS, Funkenstein HH, Smith LA, Hebert LE, Wetle TT, Hennekens CH, Branch LG, Chown M, Taylor JO (1990) Estimated prevalence of Alzheimer's disease in the United States. Milbank Quart 68:267–289

Hennekens CH, Buring JE (1987) Epidemiology in medicine. Little Brown, Boston

MacMahon B, Trichopoulos D (1996) Epidemiology principles and methods. Little Brown, Boston

Rose G (1992) The strategy of preventive medicine. Oxford, London

Possibilities for Secondary Prevention of Alzheimer's Disease

*I. Skoog**

Summary

The aim of secondary prevention is to detect a disease early, when it is asymptomatic, and by treatment prevent it from progressing into a serious outcome. Several criteria must be fulfilled before a secondary prevention programme can start. First, the disease has to have a preclinical phase that is possible to detect, it should be common enough to warrant a search for its latent stages, and the consequences of the untreated condition must be substantial. Second, an effective screening test must exist that is acceptable to the population and suitable for routine application. Third, there must be enough resources to do a diagnostic workup in those patients with a positive screen. Finally, an effective therapy must exist that is more beneficial at the presymptomatic than at the symptomatic phase.

Alzheimer's disease has a preclinical phase characterized by a large number of cognitive, psychiatric, behavioral and subcortical symptoms. However, there is a large overlap with normal aging, which makes screening difficult. The screening instruments presently used are mainly directed towards the cognitive symptoms of dementia and are not specific for Alzheimer's disease. Early therapeutic interventions in Alzheimer's disease are not possible at present as no specific treatment exists that could reverse or delay the disease process. However, secondary prevention may be directed towards comorbid conditions that may increase the possibility that individuals with Alzheimer's disease pathology express a dementia syndrome. If drugs acting directly against the neuronal damage in Alzheimer's disease are successful, the role of secondary prevention of Alzheimer's disease may change dramatically.

* Institute of Clinical Neuroscience, Department of Psychiatry, Sahlgrenska University Hospital, Göteborg University, Göteborg, Sweden.
Address for correspondence:
Ingmar Skoog, MD, PhD, Department of Psychiatry, Sahlgrenska, Sahlgrenska University Hospital, SE-413 45 Göteborg, Sweden, Telephone: +4 63 13 42 12 89, Fax: +46 31 82 81 63,
e-mail: Ingmar.Skoog@psychiat.gu.se.

R. Mayeux / Y. Christen (Eds.)
Epidemiology of Alzheimer's Disease:
From Gene to Prevention

Prevention

Prevention is often classified into several levels, depending on when interventions are instituted in relation to the clinical symptoms of the disorder (Fig. 1). The aim of primary prevention is to preserve health by removing the precipitating causes and determinants of the disease. In epidemiological terms, the aim of primary prevention is to reduce the incidence of disease by eliminating the causes or main risk factors (Last 1988).

The aim of secondary prevention is to prevent the disease from progressing into a serious outcome by means of early detection followed by definite treatment. In epidemiological terms, the aim of secondary prevention is to reduce the prevalence of the disease.

Several criteria must be fulfilled before a secondary prevention programme can start (Wallace and Everett 1992; Thomas 1992; Wilson and Jungner 1968). These can be divided into criteria related to the disease, the screening, the treatment and the evaluation.

Considerations related to the disease are that the disorder should be common enough to warrant a search for its latent stages, because screening for very rare diseases may result in unacceptable cost-benefit ratios. Second, the disorder should have a preclinical phase that is possible to detect. Ideally, the preclinical phase should be long. Finally, the consequences of the untreated condition must be substantial.

Considerations related to the screening procedure include the existence of an effective screening test, with acceptable sensitivity, specificity and predictive

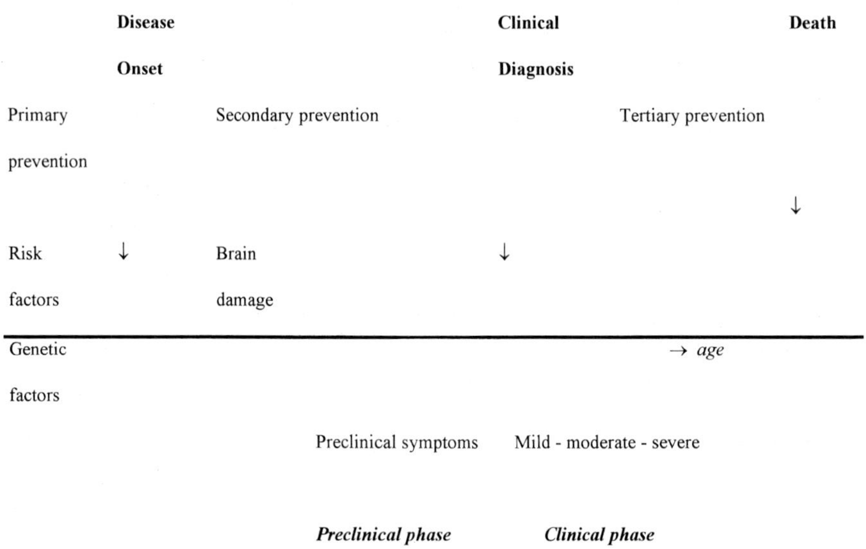

Fig. 1. Progression of Alzheimer's disease

value. The screening test should be acceptable to the population and suitable for routine application. The consequences of a false positive or a false negative test should be acceptable. Finally, there must be enough resources to do a diagnostic work-up in those patients with a positive screen.

Considerations regarding treatment are that an effective therapy must exist that is more beneficial when applied to the presymptomatic than to the symptomatic phase.

In this chapter, these criteria will be presented in more detail in relation to Alzheimer's disease. At present, several of the criteria are not fulfilled for Alzheimer's disease, such as the lack of effective screening instruments and definite treatment. If second generation drugs for Alzheimer's disease, acting directly against the neuronal damage, are successful, the role for secondary prevention of Alzheimer's disease may change dramatically.

The Disease

The Disease Should be Common Enough to Warrant a Search for its Latent Stages

Screening for very rare diseases in the general population will result in a high proportion of false positive tests, leading to unacceptable costs for society and unnecessary trauma for the individual. Therefore, target populations at high risk of the disease are often identified (Thomas 1992). Examples of populations at increased risk for Alzheimer's disease are the age group above age 75–80, individuals with a family history of dementia, individuals with low education, individuals homozygotic for the apoE ε4 allele, individuals with Down's syndrome, individuals with poor performance on cognitive testing, individuals with a history of severe head trauma, families with autosomal dominant mutations (e.g., in the presenilin-1 gene) and individuals with vascular disorders (e.g., white matter lesions or hypertension). The selection of high risk populations requires ethical consideration as it may be a psychological trauma to be selected. Genetic testing in asymptomatic individuals to identify groups at high risk of developing Alzheimer's disease is not warranted, except for rare autosomal dominant early-onset families (Post et al. 1997). The presence of an ε4 allele of APOE, and especially ε4 homozygosity, increases the lifetime risk for developing Alzheimer's disease but it is not sufficient to predict disease in asymptomatic individuals, and a large proportion of individuals with this phenotype will never develop the disease.

The Consequences of the Untreated Condition Must be Substantial

This criterion is relevant for Alzheimer's disease, which is a chronic disorder with a slowly progressive course. During the course of the disease, the patient's functions in daily living inevitably deteriorate. Alzheimer's disease is therefore the most important cause of institutionalization in the very elderly (Skoog et al. 1993; Fratiglioni et al. 1994).

Survival is reduced in Alzheimer's disease, and it is considered to be the fourth or fifth most common cause of death in Western society. The influence of dementia on survival at high ages is substantial because of its high prevalence. Katzman et al. (1994) reported a population attributable risk (PAR) for death in Alzheimer's disease and vascular dementia of 5 % in the age group 65–74 years and 21 % in those above age 75. In 85-year-olds, Aevarsson et al. (1998) reported a PAR for death in Alzheimer's disease and vascular dementia of 31 % in men and 50 % in women.

The Disease Should Have a Preclinical Phase

Alzheimer's disease is generally believed to have a slowly progressive course with an incipient onset (McKhann et al. 1984). Longitudinal studies show that its preclinical phase starts many years, or even decades, before it becomes clinically manifest. These studies report that the preclinical phase is mainly characterized by impairments in cognitive functions, such as memory, language, spatial orientation, immediate auditory attention, concentration and psychomotor speed (Ritchie et al. 1996; Dartigues et al. 1997; Masur et al. 1994; Jacobs et al. 1995; Persson et al. 1991; Persson and Skoog 1992; Aevarsson 1998). The symptoms noted during this phase are generally subtle and difficult to distinguish from normality at an individual level. The early phase also includes a large number of psychiatric manifestations, such as visual hallucinations, paranoid symptoms, compulsions (Aevarsson 1998) and depressed mood (Devanand et al. 1996). Behavioural symptoms during this phase involve symptoms of inhibition or retardation (Persson et al. 1991; Verhey 1993; Aevarsson 1998) as well as of decreased inhibition (Aevarsson 1998). Finally, an increased frequency of extrapyramidal signs has been noted (Richards et al. 1993). It is believed that these early symptoms reflect degeneration in certain areas of the brain.

Screening

A major part of secondary prevention is screening. The purpose of screening is to detect individuals with asymptomatic (latent) disease who can be effectively treated (Wallace and Everett 1992). A prerequisite for secondary prevention is, therefore, the existence of an effective screening test, with an acceptable high sensitivity, specificity and predictive value.

Sensitivity

Sensitivity is the proportion of the patients with the disease (i.e., false negatives and true positives) who are classified as diseased with the test, expressed as:

Sensitivity = [true positives/(true positives + false negatives)] × 100

True positives are individuals with the disease whose test results are positive. False negatives are individuals whose test results are negative despite the fact that they have the disease (Wallace and Everett 1992). Sensitivity is decreased by the proportion of cases missed by the test (false negatives). The number of patients with the disease who will be missed (false negatives) increases as the sensitivity of the test decreases. As the sensitivity increases, so do the number of false positives in most cases.

Specificity

Specificity is the proportion of true healthy individuals (i.e., false positives and true negatives) who are classified as healthy, expressed as:

Specificity = [true negatives/(false positives + true negatives)] × 100

Specificity is decreased by the proportion of healthy individuals who have a positive test result (false positives). As the specificity of the test decreases, the number of people that will erroneously be considered to have the disease (false positives) increases.

Sensitivity and specificity are generally inversely related. As sensitivity increases, specificity decreases, and vice versa.

The Positive Predictive Value

The positive predictive value is the proportion of individuals with a positive test (i.e., true positives and false positives) who actually have the disease, expressed as:

Positive predictive value = [true positives/(true positives + false positives)] × 100

The positive predictive value is decreased by the proportion of non-cases found to be positive (false positives). As the positive predictive value of the test decreases, the proportion of healthy people among those with a positive screen (false positives) increases.

Application of Screening Instruments in Different Types of Samples

Sensitivity, specificity and positive predictive values for different screening instruments are in general applicable only to similar populations and circumstances in which they were performed (Wallace and Everett 1992; Ritchie 1988). At any given sensitivity and specificity, the positive predictive value is directly related to the prevalence of the disease (Galen and Gambino 1975), i.e., if the prevalence is high, the positive predictive value will also be high, and it will

Table 1. Positive predictive value in populations with different prevalences of the disease

Prevalence	Sensitivity 95 % Specificity 95 %	Sensitivity 87 % Specificity 92 %	Sensitivity 80 % Specificity 80 %	Sensitivity 50 % Specificity 50 %
1 %	19 %	10 %	4 %	1 %
5 %	50 %	36 %	17 %	5 %
10 %	68 %	55 %	31 %	10 %
20 %	82 %	73 %	50 %	20 %
75 %	95 %	97 %	92 %	75 %

decline if the prevalence of the disease declines. This is illustrated in Table 1. For example, if we have a test with a high sensitivity (e.g., 95 %) and high specificity (e.g., 95 %), and we assume that the prevalence of dementia is 1 %, then only one of five individuals with a positive test will actually have the disease. Eighty percent will have a false positive test. Thus, a high sensitivity of a test applied in a population with a low prevalence of the disease will result in a high number of false positives. On the other hand, when the prevalence of the disease is high, positive predictive value will be high. In summary, more false-negative test results occur if the disease is common, and more false positive tests occur if the disease is rare (Thomas 1992).

Instruments developed and validated on patient samples may thus not have the same sensitivity and specificity when applied to unselected population samples (Ritchie 1988), where secondary prevention is supposed to be performed. Most tests and biological markers for Alzheimer's disease are tested and developed in clinical settings, where the proportion of Alzheimer's disease is high. Thus, the positive predictive value in these settings is deemed to be high, as may be seen in Table 1. One example of this is the finding that the presence of the apoE ε4 allele in demented patients with suspected Alzheimer's disease in special evaluation units has a high predictive value for the neuropathologic diagnosis of Alzheimer's disease (Saunders et al. 1996). In these units, the prevalence of Alzheimer's disease at autopsy was high, about 85 %. In more unselected populations, the positive predictive value is probably considerably lower.

One should also consider that the first screening (prevalence screen) has a higher positive predictive value than the second screening (incidence screen), because the first screening includes all cases irrespective of onset whereas the second screening includes only new cases (Fletcher et al. 1996).

Screening for Alzheimer's Disease

Although there is a preclinical phase of Alzheimer's disease, there is a large overlap in symptomatology between non-demented individuals who later develop dementia (subclinical cases) and those who do not, and between those who develop Alzheimer's disease and vascular dementia. At present no effective and specific screening test for Alzheimer's disease exists, but several short instruments for the detection of the cognitive symptoms of dementia are in use. These tests may detect dementia per se, but they are not specific for Alzheimer's disease and those detected have to go through an extensive work-up to decide whether they have dementia or not and, if so, if they have Alzheimer's disease or some other type of dementia. Furthermore, these cognitive tests are effective in screening for moderate to severe dementia but less effective in finding cases with mild or preclinical dementia.

Furthermore, the selection of a cut-off score is difficult because the dimensional rather than categorical character makes subclinical and mild dementia often difficult to separate from normal aging (Brayne and Calloway 1989; Henderson and Huppert 1984; Mowry and Burvill 1988). It is possible that screening tests that take the individual's previous intellectual level into consideration (e.g., by obtaining information from key informants or by following the patients over time) may be more effective in screening for mild or preclinical dementia.

The most widely used instrument to screen for the cognitive symptoms of dementia is the Mini-Mental State Examination (MMSE; Folstein et al. 1975). Its maximum test score is 30. The traditional cut-off score of 23/24 is regarded to be compatible with a clinical diagnosis of moderate to severe dementia. As the MMSE is the most widely used and validated screening instrument for dementia, it will be used as an example of a cognitive screening instrument in this review. In common with other similar screening instruments, the MMSE detects most cases of moderate to severe dementia but about half of the cases with mild dementia are screened negative (Kay et al. 1985; Aevarsson 1998).

In cross-sectional population studies, a cut-off score of 23/24 in the MMSE has been shown to have acceptable sensitivity and specificity for the detection of prevalent cases of dementia (O'Connor et al. 1989; Grut et al. 1993; Aevarsson 1998), generally in the range of 80–90 %. These figures are in relation to dementia in general, and sensitivity and specificity are probably much lower in mild or subclinical dementia, which are the target populations for secondary prevention. Sensitivity, specificity and positive predictive value for different cut-off scores of the MMSE are shown in Table 2. In line with most screening instruments for the

Table 2. Sensitivity, specificity and positive predictive values (PPV) for different cut-off points on the MMSE. The Kungsholmen Study[a]

Cut-off	Sensitivity	Specificity	PPV
17/18	54	98	91
18/19	58	98	85
19/20	61	98	84
20/21	66	97	82
21/22	71	96	77
22/23	79	94	71
23/24	87	92	68
24/25	90	86	57
25/26	94	77	44
26/27	97	62	34
27/28	100	41	26

[a] Grut et al. 1993.

Table 3. Proportion of vascular dementia using different criteria[a]

N = 85	%
DSM-IV	76
ICD-10	33
NINDS-AIREN	14
Chui criteria	27

[a] Wetterling et al. (1996).

cognitive symptoms of dementia, performance on the MMSE is influenced be educational level (Crum et al. 1993; Jacqmin-Gadda et al. 1997; Ylikoski et al. 1992).

Another problem in secondary prevention of Alzheimer's disease is the definition of a true positive case. The most often used criteria for the clinical diagnosis of Alzheimer's disease are those of the NINCDS-ADRDA (McKhann et al. 1984), which mainly represent diagnosis by exclusion and do not specify how to diagnose patients with concomitant vascular diseases. The agreement between the NINCDS-ADRDA criteria and neuropathological diagnosis of Alzheimer's disease has been reported to be 80–90 % (Jellinger 1996; Mendez et al. 1992). However, these correlations emanate from specialized academic centers and are based on patients followed for several years. The accuracy rate in the earlier stages of the disease and in large-scale prevention programs is not known.

The main diagnostic problem is to distinguish Alzheimer's disease from vascular dementia Alzheimer's disease may sometimes have a course suggestive of vascular dementia, and vascular dementia may have a course suggestive of Alzheimer's disease (Erkinjuntti and Sulkava 1991; Fischer et al. 1990). Alzheimer's disease may be underdiagnosed in persons with cerebral infarcts as neither clinical nor pathological evidence of cerebrovascular disease means that it caused the dementia. However, Alzheimer's disease may also be overdiagnosed as many infarctions are clinically silent and infarcts in cases of typical Alzheimer's disease may be dismissed as being irrelevant. Depending on the criteria used, the proportion of demented individuals diagnosed as Alzheimer's disease or vascular dementia may differ considerably (Skoog et al. 1993; Amar et al. 1996; Wetterling et al. 1996), as may be seen in Table 3.

Acceptability

A screening test has to be acceptable to those screened with regard to safety, pain, other discomfort, adverse consequences, esthetic and cultural barriers, the costs and efforts. If the test is not acceptable for these reasons, people may not agree to be screened (Thomas 1992).

No biological marker exists for Alzheimer's disease today. Analysis of cerebrospinal fluid (CSF) shows a markedly decreased level of β-amyloid Aβ(1–42) (Motter et al. 1995) and an increased level of tau protein (Blennow et al. 1995; Skoog et al. 1995) in Alzheimer's disease. Even if these biochemical markers should be effective in identifying very early Alzheimer's disease in unselected populations, a lumbar puncture will probably not be acceptable as a general screening instrument for Alzheimer's disease. However, acceptability will increase if effective early therapies exist.

Suitability

The test must also be acceptable to the clinicians who are supposed to administer it. It must thus be easy and possible to administer to the people in the target population (Thomas 1992). The time to administer it should be short. The formal qualifications needed for the staff that administer it should be as small as possible. Ideally, special equipment and special resources should be kept at a minimum, and the test should be administered at the usual appointment and not at an extra session. The preparation of patients should be minimal and the costs of screening and subsequent evaluations minimal. Most of these criteria apply to the short screening instruments used to detect dementia at present. However, even if the test is simple to administer, the work-up for those screened positive may be costly and exhaustive.

The Consequences of a False Positive Test

A false positive test is a false alarm. The consequences of this for the individual, the medical care system, and the screening program must be considered before a screening test and its cut-off score against normality is chosen (Thomas 1992). A test with a high sensitivity will detect more of the cases, but will also lead to more false positive cases.

It is the falsely screened who have to pay for the successful screening and treatment of the true positive. For the individual, a false positive test will lead to unnecessary psychological trauma and inconvenience. The positively screened individual may get a negative labeling, i.e., a negative psychological reaction because of the test result (Fletcher et al. 1996). For example, if a test for cognitive function is used for the screening of Alzheimer's disease, the falsely screened positive will have a label of being cognitively impaired even if the work-up shows that he does not have Alzheimer's disease, or even dementia. If the test leads to auxillary investigations, it will take unnecessary time for the falsely screened and the examinations may be exhaustive and painful. It has to be decided how much of this the erroneously screened individual will have to bear. When deciding whether a secondary prevention program should start, one should calculate the ratio of false positives, not only for every true positive, but for every true positive who is successfully treated, and decide whether this ratio is acceptable.

There Must be Resources for a Diagnostic Work-Up in Those who had a Positive Screen

It has to be decided whether there are sufficient facilities and personnel to provide the necessary diagnostic test to determine whether those screened positive actually have the disease. It is necessary to decide the cost-benefits and if there is someone who will pay the costs. One must also consider the reactions from physicians who will have a large number of healthy people referred to them for diagnostic evaluation.

In Alzheimer's disease, a complete work-up in those screened positive includes careful history-taking, neurological, psychiatric and physical examinations, interview with a close informant, brain imaging, a chest X-ray, and biochemical screening including vitamin B_{12} level, a thyroid function test and, in selected cases, a cerebrospinal fluid examination (Katzmann 1986). These procedures are necessary to exclude other causes of dementia (such as hypothyroidism, vitamin B_{12} deficiency, brain tumors, normal pressure hydrocephalus, subdural hematoma or cerebrovascular disease) and have generally not been possible to perform in large scale studies such as screening programs.

The Consequences of a False Negative Test

A false negative test may give a false sense of security, and the disease may then progress to a noncurable stage (Thomas 1992). For the screening of Alzheimer's disease and cognitive impairment, this may be the case if there is a treatable secondary form of dementia (e.g., a brain tumour) that progresses to an uncurable stage. This scenario could have legal implications, particularly if a more sensitive test, or a more sensitive cut-off score, could have been used. In the future, if more effective treatments for Alzheimer's disease are introduced, the question of false negatives will be even more important.

An Effective Therapy Must Exist

Current Possibilities

Early therapeutic interventions and secondary prevention in cases of Alzheimer's disease are not possible at present because no specific treatment exists that could reverse or delay the disease process. The present treatments with first generation drugs for Alzheimer's disease (i.e., acetylcholine esterase inhibitors, such as tacrine and donepezil), which slightly improve dementia symptoms by preventing the breakdown of acetylcholine, are only symptomatic. It is not clear whether these drugs, if introduced at the preclinical phase, could delay the onset of clinical symptoms of dementia.

Secondary prevention of dementia may at present also include measures to identify "reversible" contributing causes of the clinical symptoms of Alzheimer's disease, such as brain tumors, subdural hematomas, thyroid disease, depression, normal pressure hydrocephalus, and vascular disorders. With regard to cerebrovascular disorders, many infarcts are clinically silent. It was recently reported that concomitant cerebrovascular diseases increase the possibility that individuals with Alzheimer's disease pathology will express a dementia syndrome (Snowdon et al. 1997). Thus, treatment of these contributing causes may actually reverse the clinical symptoms of Alzheimer's disease. Vascular disorders are common in elderly populations. Their etiologic fraction for the clinical expression of Alzheimer's disease may thus be high. Some prospective intervention studies are now underway to test the possibility that treatment of hypertension may prevent Alzheimer's disease.

Future Possibilities

If second generation Alzheimer's disease drugs, acting directly against the neuronal damage, are successful, the role for secondary prevention of Alzheimer's disease may change dramatically. Other possibilities for treatment in the future may include the use of estrogens (Tang et al. 1996), anti-inflammatory drugs (McGeer and McGeer 1995; Breitner et al. 1995), antioxidants (such as selegiline and α-tocopherol; Sano et al. 1997), antihypertensive drugs (such as ACE-inhibitors; Skoog 1997), gangliosides and growth factors. Trials are now underway to test several of these compounds.

Another requirement, if secondary prevention should be considered, is that the treatment should be more beneficial when applied to the presymptomatic than to the symptomatic phase. However, at present, there is no evidence of an anti-dementia drug that is more effective at the preclinical than at the clinical phase, although intuitively it seems likely that early treatment would be beneficial in Alzheimer's disease.

Evaluation of Secondary Prevention

Program evaluation should be considered when the program is being planned. Some lessons applicable to Alzheimer's disease could be learned from secondary prevention of other chronic disorders.

Evaluation of the effectiveness of secondary prevention should consider three levels. First, one must evaluate whether treatment in presymptomatic individuals who are screened positive is beneficial. This could be done by means of randomized double-blind clinical trials. Second, one must evaluate whether treatment at the subclinical stage is more effective than treatment after symptom onset. Finally, one must evaluate whether the whole program (including screening and treatment) is effective. Some pitfalls exist for the last two levels that may lead to misleading results regarding a screening program's value (Wallace and Everett 1992).

One of these occurs when treatment at the subclinical stage is evaluated against treatment after symptom onset by comparing treatment response in these groups (Thomas 1992). By definition those detected at screening more often have a less advanced disorder. However, these mild cases detected at screening may not have a similar course as those detected after symptom onset. For example, a large proportion of those with subclinical cognitive deterioration do not progress to manifest Alzheimer's disease, but the great majority of cases with manifest Alzheimer dementia progress to a more severe form. Thus, if treatment response for cases detected at screening is compared to cases detected after symptom onset and measured as the progression of clinical symptoms, the impression may be that early treatment is more beneficial than late treatment even if there is no treatment response at all.

As Alzheimer's disease is associated with reduced survival, mortality could be another measure used to evaluate the screening program. However, the comparison of survival rates, or time to death, between cases detected at screening and cases detected by other means may give rise to the so-called lead time bias (Thomas 1992). This is when the identification of a disorder by a screening test during its presymptomatic stage increases the duration of the disorder just because the disease is diagnosed earlier, without changing the ultimate outcome.

Disorders such as Alzheimer's disease progress at varying rates. Length bias sampling occurs when there is a correlation between the duration of the presymptomatic phase and the course of the symptomatic phase (Thomas 1992). If the mild form of the disease has a longer presymptomatic phase, it will be more often detected at screening than the more severe forms. Therefore, compared to symptomatic cases, a higher proportion of dementias detected at screening will be slowly progressive, so the patient's survival from time of detection will tend to be longer, even if early detection does not result in a prolongation of time-to-death. If so, the screening test and the following treatment may appear falsely beneficial. Further on, some cases will have such a slow progression, or even be stationary, that they would never have progressed to a clinical stage. These cases will seem to have responded to treatment, although the treatment was unnecessary.

References

Aevarsson O (1998) Dementia and ageing. An epidemiological study of the detection, preclinical phase, course and prognosis of dementia at age 85 to 88 (Dissertation). Gothenburg University. Gothenburg

Aevarsson O, Svanborg A, Skoog I (1998) Seven-year survival after age 85. Relation to Alzheimer's disease and vascular dementia. Arch Neurol, 55, 1226–1232

Amar K, Wilcock GK, Scott M (1996) The diagnosis of vascular dementia in the light of the new criteria. Age Ageing 25:51–55

Blennow K, Vanmechelen E, Wallin A (1995) Tau protein in cerebrospinal fluid: a biochemical diagnostic marker for axonal degeneration in Alzheimer's disease? Mol Chem Neuropathol 26:231–245

Brayne C, Calloway P (1989) An epidemiological study of dementia in a rural population of elderly women. Br J Psychiat 155:214–219

Breitner JCS, Welsh KA, Helms MJ, Gaskell PC, Gau BA, Roses AD, Pericak-Vance MA, Saunders AM (1995) Delayed onset of Alzheimer's disease with non-steroidal anti-inflammatory and histamine H2 blocking drugs. Neurobiol Aging 16:523–530

Crum RM, Anthony JC, Bassett SS, Folstein MF (1993) Population-based norms for the Mini-Mental State Examination by age and educational level. JAMA 269:2386–2391

Dartigues JF, Commenges D, Letenneur L, Barberger-Gateau P, Gilleron V, Fabrigoule C, Mazaux JM, Orgogozo JM, Salamon R (1997) Cognitive predictors of dementia in elderly community residents. Neuroepidemiology 16:29–39

Devanand DP, Sano M, Tang MX, Taylor S, Gurland BJ, Wilder D, Stern Y, Mayeux R (1996) Depressed mood and the incidence of Alzheimer's disease in the elderly living in the community. Arch Gen Psychiat 53:175–182

Erkinjuntti T, Sulkava R (1991) Diagnosis of multi-infarct dementia. Alzheimer Dis Assoc Disord 5:112–121

Fischer P, Gatterer G, Marterer A, Simanyi M, Danielczyk W (1990) Course characteristics in the differentiation of dementia of the Alzheimer type and multi-infarct dementia. Acta Psychiatr Scand 81:551–553

Fletcher RH, Fletcher SW, Wagner EH (1996) Clinical epidemiology. The essentials. Third Edition. Williams & Williams, Baltimore

Folstein MF, Folstein SE, McHugh PR (1975) "Mini-mental state." A practical method for grading the cognitive state of patients for the clinician. J Psychiatr Res 12:189–198

Fratiglioni L, Forsell Y, Torres HA, Winblad B (1994) Severity of dementia and institutionalization in the elderly: Prevalence data from an urban area in Sweden. Neuroepidemiology 13:79–88

Galen RS, Gambino SR (1975) Beyond normality: the predictive value and efficiency of medical diagnosis. John Wiley. New York

Grut M, Fratiglioni L, Viitanen M, Winblad B (1993) Accuracy of the Mini-Mental Status Examination as a screening test for dementia in a Swedish elderly population. Acta Neurol Scand 87:312–317

Henderson AS, Huppert FA (1984) The problem of mild dementia. Psychol Med 14:5–11

Jacobs DM, Sano M, Dooneief G, Marder K, Bell KL, Stern Y (1995) Neuropsychological detection and characterization of preclinical Alzheimer's disease. Neurology 45:957–962

Jacqmin-Gadda H, Fabrigoule C, Commenges D, Dartigues J-F (1997) A 5-year longitudinal study of the Mini-Mental State Examination in normal aging. Am J Epidemiol 145:498–506

Jellinger KA (1996) Diagnostic accuracy of Alzheimer's disease: a clinicopathological study. Acta Neuropathol 91:219–220

Katzman R. Alzheimer's disease (1986) New Engl J Med 314:964–973

Katzman R, Hill LR, Yu ESH, Wang Z-Y, Booth A, Salmon DP, Liu WT, Qu GY, Zhang M (1994) The malignancy of dementia. Predictors of mortality in clinically diagnosed dementia in a population survey of Shanghai, China. Arch Neurol 51:1220–1225

Kay DWK, Henderson AS, Scott R, Wilson J, Rickwood D, Grayson DA (1985) Dementia and depression among the elderly living in the Hobart community: the effect of the diagnostic criteria on the prevalence rates. Psychol Med 15:771–788

Last JM (1988) A dictionary of epidemiology. Second edition. Oxford University Press, New York

Masur DM, Sliwinski M, Lipton RB, Blau AD, Crystal HA (1994) Neuropsychological prediction of dementia and the absence of dementia in healthy elderly persons. Neurology 44:1427–1432

McGeer PL, McGeer EG (1995) The inflammatory response system of the brain: implications for therapy of Alzheimer and other neurodegenerative diseases. Brain Res Rev 21:195–218

McKhann G, Drachman D, Folstein M, Katzman R, Price D, Stadlan EM (1984) Clinical diagnosis of Alzheimer's disease: report of the NINCDS-ADRDA Work Group under the auspices of Department of Health and Human Services task force on Alzheimer's disease. Neurology 34:939–44

Mendez MF, Mastri AR, Sung JH, Frey WH (1992) Clinically diagnosed Alzheimer disease: neuropathologic findings in 650 cases. Alzheimer Dis Assoc Disord 6:35–43

Motter R, Vigo-Pelfrey C, Kholodenko D, Barbour R, Johnson-Wood K, Galasko D, Chang L, Miller B, Clark C, Green R, Olson D, Southwick P, Wolfert R, Munroe B, Lieberburg I, Seat P, Schenk D (1995) Reduction of β-amyloid $peptide_{42}$ in the cerebrospinal fluid of patients with Alzheimer's disease. Ann Neurol 38:643–648

Mowry BJ, Burvill PW (1988) A study of mild dementia in the community using a wide range of diagnostic criteria. Br J Psychiat 153:328–334

O'Connor DW, Pollitt PA, Treasure FP, Brooks CPB, Reiss BB (1989) The influence of education, social class and sex on Mini-Mental State scores. Psychol Med 19:771–776

Persson G, Skoog (1992) Subclinical dementia: Relevance of cognitive and affective symptoms and signs. A nine year prospective study. J Geriatr Psychiat Neurol 5:172–178

Persson G, Berg S, Nilsson L, Svanborg A (1991) Subclinical dementia. Relation to cognition, personality and psychopathology: a nine-year prospective study. Int J Geriatr Psychiat 6:239–247

Post SG, Whitehouse PJ, Binstock RH, Bird TD, Eckert SK, Farrer LA, Fleck LM, Gaines AD, Juengst ET, Karlinsky H, Miles S, Murray TH, Quaid KA, Relkin NR, Roses AD, St George-Hyslop PH, Sachs GA, Steinbock B, Truschke EF, Zinn AB (1997) The clinical introduction of genetic testing for Alzheimer's disease. An ethical perspective. JAMA 277:832–836

Richards M, Stern Y, Mayeux R (1993) Subtle extrapyramidal signs can predict the development of dementia in elderly individuals. Neurology 43:2184–2188

Ritchie K (1988) The screening of cognitive impairment in the elderly: A critical review of current methods. J Clin Epidemiol 41:635–643

Ritchie K, Leibovici D, Ledésert B, Touchon J (1996) A typology of sub-clinical senescent cognitive disorders. Br J Psychiat 168:470–476

Sano M, Ernesto C, Thomas RG, Klauber MR, Schafer K, Grundman M, Woodbury P, Growdon J, Cotman CW, Pfeiffer E, Schneider LS, Thal LJ (1997) A controlled trial of selegiline, alpha-tocopherol, or both as treatment for Alzheimer's disease. New Engl J Med 336:1216–1222

Saunders AM, Hulette O, Welsh-Bohmer KA, Schmechel DE, Crain B, Burke JR, Alberts MJ, Strittmatter WJ, Breitner JC, Rosenberg C, Scott SV, Gaskell PC Jr., Pericak-Vance MA, Roses AD (1996) Specificity, sensitivity, and predictive value of apolipoprotein-E genotyping for sporadic Alzheimer's disease. Lancet 348:90–93

Skoog I (1997) Blood pressure and dementia. A review. Biomed Pharmacother 5:367–375

Skoog I, Nilsson L, Palmertz B, Andreasson L-A, Svanborg A (1993) A population-based study of dementia in 85-year-olds. New Engl J Med 328:153–158

Skoog I, Vanmechelen E, Andreasson L-A, Palmertz B, Davidsson P, Hesse C, Blennow K (1995) A population-based study of tau protein and ubiquitin in cerebrospinal fluid in 85-year-olds: relation to severity of dementia and cerebral atrophy, but not to the apolipoprotein E4 allele. Neurodegeneration 4:433–442

Snowdon DA, Greiner LH, Mortimer JA, Riley KP, Greiner PA, Markesbery WR (1997) Brain infarction and the clinical expression of Alzheimer disease. The Nun Study. JAMA 277:813–817

Tang M-X, Jacobs D, Stern Y, Marder K, Scofield P, Gurland B, Andrews H, Mayeux R (1996) Effect of oestrogen during menopause on risk and age at onset of Alzheimer's disease. Lancet 348:429–432

Thomas DB (1992) Cancer. In: Last JM, Wallace RB (eds) Maxcy-Rosenau-Last. Public Health & Preventive Medicine. Appleton & Lange, East Norwalk, Connecticut, pp 811–826

Verhey FRJ (1993) Dementia, depression and forgetfulness. Clinical studies of the early diagnosis and the differential diagnosis of dementia. (Thesis). University of Maastricht

Wallace RB, Everett GD (1992) Prevention of chronic illness. In: Last JM, Wallace RB (eds). Maxcy-Rosenau-Last. Public Health & Preventive Medicine. Appleton & Lange, East Norwalk, Connecticut, pp 805–810

Wetterling T, Kanitz R-D, Borgis K-J (1996) Comparison of different diagnostic criteria for vascular dementia (ADDTC, DSM-IV, ICD-10, NINDS-AIREN). Stroke 27:30–36

Wilson JMG, Jungner G (1968) Principles and practice of screening for disease. Publ Health Pap No34. WHO, Geneva

Ylikoski R, Erkinjuntti T, Sulkava R, Juva K, Tilvis R, Valvanne J (1992) Correction for age, education and other demographic variables in the use of the Mini Mental State Examination in Finland. Acta Neurol Scand 85:391–396

Subject Index

Printing: Saladruck, Berlin
Binding: Buchbinderei Lüderitz & Bauer, Berlin